Everyday
Gluten-Free

pil

Publications International, Ltd.

Pictured on the front cover *(clockwise from top left):* Classic Brownies *(page 176)*, Pesto Zoodles & Potatoes *(page 148)*, Blueberry Coconut Flour Muffins *(page 161)* and Spinach & Mushroom Cauliflower Pizza *(page 70)*.

Pictured on the back cover *(top to bottom):* Herbed Pork with Potatoes & Green Beans *(page 118)* and Cauliflower Parmesan *(page 122)*.

Photographs and art on front cover and pages 8, 10, 71, 160 and 177 copyright © Shutterstock.com.

ISBN: 978-1-63938-052-7

Manufactured in China.

8 7 6 5 4 3 2 1

Microwave Cooking: Microwave ovens vary in wattage. Use the cooking times as guidelines and check for doneness before adding more time.

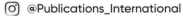

Let's get social!
@Publications_International
@PublicationsInternational
www.pilbooks.com

contents

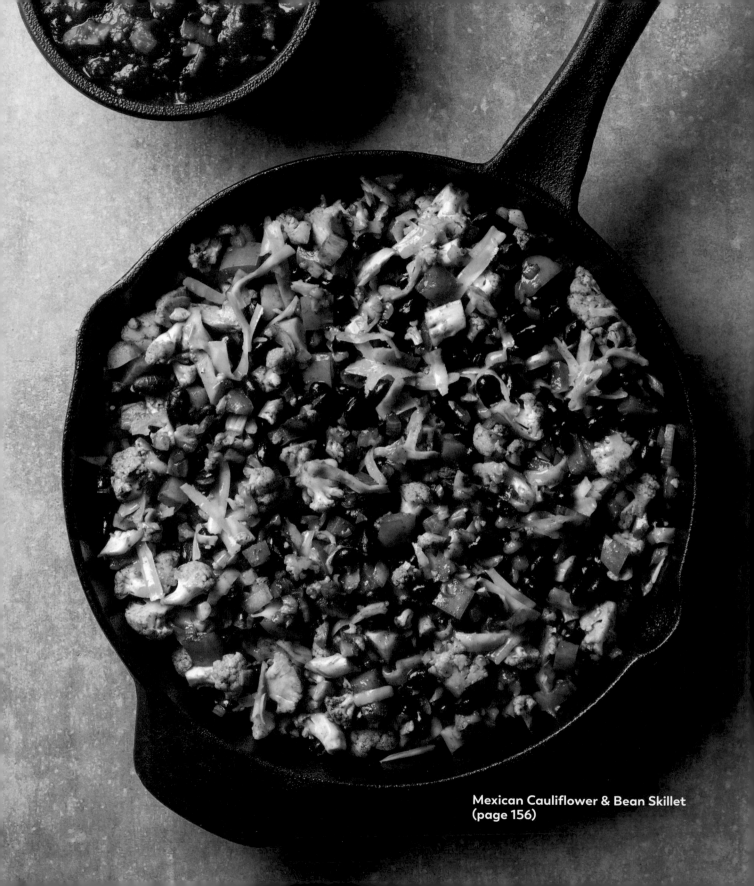

Mexican Cauliflower & Bean Skillet
(page 156)

introduction

What Is Gluten Anyway?

It's not just wheat. Gluten is a protein that is found naturally in wheat, rye and barley. Gluten gives structure to the baked goods we know and love. Without it, or something to replace it, bread and cake would be sad little puddles or piles of crumbs. When yeast, baking powder or other leavening agents produce bubbles in a dough or a batter, that air is trapped by the stretchy gluten network and the baked product rises and becomes light.

Legend has it that gluten was discovered by 7th century Buddhist monks who were trying to find something to replace the texture and savor of meat in their vegetarian diets. They found that when they submerged dough made with wheat flour in water, the starch washed away. What was left behind was a gummy mass with an almost meatlike texture—gluten. Today gluten is still used to make seitan, mock duck and other meat replacement products.

Celiac Disease, Gluten Intolerance and Wheat Allergies

There are many reasons people choose to avoid gluten and many forms of gluten intolerance. Celiac disease is one of the most serious. In the 1% of Americans diagnosed with this autoimmune disorder, exposure to even small amounts of gluten can cause intestinal damage and result in symptoms from fatigue to anemia and bone disease. It is estimated that millions more may have undiagnosed celiac disease—as many as 1 out of every 133 Americans.

Whether you have celiac disease or another form of gluten intolerance it's good to understand the distinction. Celiac disease is a very specific condition in which exposure to gluten causes the villi, or small hairlike projections from the small intestine, to become atrophied. The purpose of these villi and the spaces between them is to let the body absorb nutrients and keep out toxins. With celiac disease, the immune system sees fragments of gluten as toxins and reacts by attacking not only the gluten but the villi themselves. An autoimmune disease, such as celiac, occurs when the body attacks itself, mistaking normal, healthy tissue for dangerous bacteria or viruses. There are more than 80 autoimmune disorders, including rheumatoid arthritis and lupus. Most, like celiac disease, are difficult to diagnose since they present a bewildering array of symptoms.

The symptoms of celiac disease and gluten sensitivity are the same. This is not surprising since they both stem from an inability to digest gluten properly. What is surprising is that there are so many different seemingly unrelated symptoms. Most people first think of gastrointestinal distress as a sign of gluten intolerance, but symptoms may also include fatigue, weight loss, weight gain, migraine headaches, anemia and sinusitis! Because digestion is central to providing our bodies with energy, gluten intolerance and celiac disease are multi-symptomatic. Any individual may have one or many of the possible symptoms. In fact, you can have celiac disease with no symptoms at all.

It's Complicated

Just as there are many symptoms, there are many degrees of gluten sensitivity and each person's tolerance can change over time. It is possible to develop celiac disease any time in your life for any number of reasons, including enduring a stressful period. Remember, celiac is defined as damage to the intestinal villi. You could have a genetic predisposition for the disease, which only shows up under certain circumstances. Nobody knows whether what starts out as gluten intolerance can lead to celiac disease. There are also some people who are allergic to wheat itself. A classic wheat allergy is quite different from gluten intolerance. It is likely to cause the same sorts of immediate symptoms as other food allergies—itchiness, difficulty breathing and in some cases, anaphylactic shock.

On the Other Hand, It's Simple.

Millions of Americans are going gluten-free for dozens of reasons. Some have been told that they must by their doctors. Others just feel better when they stop eating gluten. Some parents feel that a gluten-free diet improves the behavior patterns of their children, including those with ADHD and autism. And there are those who just think it's trendy. Truth is, if giving up gluten didn't improve so many lives, people wouldn't be willing to make the effort. There is one caveat: if you want to try gluten-free living but haven't been tested for celiac disease, you need to be tested BEFORE you start the diet. Otherwise test results will be meaningless.

Testing, Testing, One, Two, Three

Why aren't we all tested for gluten intolerance automatically? And why does it often take years to come up with a diagnosis? Part of the problem has been lack of awareness, especially in the U.S. Some European countries require children to be tested by age five and most diagnose celiac disease in a matter of months. The average time between seeing a doctor and diagnosis in the U.S. can be more than ten years, but things are improving. Unfortunately, there is no one easy, sure-fire test to detect it.

Blood samples can determine if you produce antibodies to gluten (provided you are still consuming it for several months before blood is drawn). There are five commonly used measures. None of them, unfortunately, will prove without the shadow of a doubt that you have celiac disease. If any of them is positive, your doctor may recommend a biopsy by way of endoscopy. If this determines your villi are damaged, then there is no doubt that you have celiac disease and must go on a gluten-free diet for life.

It is possible to be genetically predisposed to celiac disease, too. If you have the disease in your family, the chances are greater that you will be affected. There is also a test for genetic markers for celiac disease. If you are lacking those genes, you won't get celiac. However, not everyone who has those genes will get sick.

Your best resource is a doctor or clinic with experience in gluten intolerance and celiac disease. Just remember—if you stop eating gluten before the tests, they will be useless. On the other hand, if you feel better when you don't eat gluten, maybe test results aren't that important.

the short list

Sensitivities differ from person to person and ingredients differ from brand to brand. Always check the label's fine print. This is an abbreviated list of some of the most commonly used items.

RED LIGHTS: (contain gluten)

- barley
- beer
- bran
- brewer's yeast
- bulgur
- cereal
- commercial baked goods
- couscous
- durum
- einkorn
- emmer
- graham
- gravies and sauces
- groats (barley or wheat)
- hydrolyzed wheat protein
- imitation seafood
- kamut
- malt vinegar
- malt, malt flavoring, malt extract
- matzo
- orzo
- pizza
- pretzels
- rye
- seitan
- semolina
- spelt
- tabbouleh
- wheat

YELLOW LIGHTS: (may contain gluten)

- artificial color*
- baking powder
- barbecue sauce
- caramel color*
- dextrins*
- emulsifiers
- flavorings
- frozen vegetables with sauce/seasonings
- hydrolyzed plant protein (HPP)
- marinades
- modified food starch*
- mustard
- nondairy creamer
- oats (see page 8)
- pasta sauce
- salad dressings
- soba noodles
- soy sauce
- vegetable broth

*These items are gluten-free if made in the U.S. or Canada.

GREEN LIGHTS: (no gluten)

- almond flour
- baking soda
- beans
- buckwheat
- carob
- carrageenan
- cellophane noodles (bean thread noodles)
- cheese
- chickpea flour (garbanzo flour, besan flour)
- corn, cornmeal
- corn grits
- corn tortillas
- dairy
- distilled alcohol
- eggs
- fruit, fresh, frozen or dried
- guar gum
- lentils
- maltodextrin
- masa harina
- meat and poultry
- millet
- mono and diglycerides
- nuts
- oils and fats
- polenta
- potatoes
- quinoa
- rice, rice flour
- rice noodles
- seafood
- sorghum flour
- soy, soy flour
- sweet rice flour (glutinous rice flour)
- tapioca
- tofu
- vegetables (fresh, canned or frozen without sauce/ seasonings)
- vinegar (except malt)
- xanthan gum

The Never-Ending Oat Controversy

Oats have been on and off the gluten-free list for years. The main problem is that most oats are processed in facilities that also handle wheat products and are contaminated for that reason. There are brands of certified gluten-free oats available (at a premium price) that have been farmed, processed and packed in a dedicated facility. These are safe for most everyone. However, there seems to be a small subset of celiac patients who have a problem with a protein present in oats.

advanced label reading

Spotting the gluten in foods is considerably easier now than ever before. Since 2004, the FDA's Food Allergy Labeling Law has required that any product containing wheat or derived from it must say so on the label. This means that many ingredients that used to be questionable, such as modified food starch and maltodextrin, must now show wheat as part of their name if they were made from it (for example, "wheat maltodextrin"). This law also applies to all eight of the most common allergens—eggs, fish, milk, peanuts, tree nuts, shellfish, soybeans and wheat. The only catch is that some sources of gluten, namely barley and rye, are NOT common allergens and don't have to be labeled. Also, you need to be aware that this ONLY applies to foods produced in the U.S. and Canada. Imports are a different matter.

Becoming a Label Detective

Going gluten-free means you may have to start bringing a magnifying glass on your shopping trips. At the very least, you will learn a great deal about the many ingredients that go into all the processed food most of us take for granted. You may even decide that paying attention to the ingredients list is a lot more relevant than some of the marketing hype that appears on the front of the package.

The red flag you're searching for is the word "wheat." If anything in the product contains, or is made from wheat, by law it must be listed as such. Next, look for any ingredients you don't recognize. Chances are you'll find a few multisyllabic words that sound like they came from the chemistry lab. You'll need to check a list of safe and unsafe ingredients to figure those out.

Soon enough, you'll recognize the most common ones that can be a problem (even if you never do learn how to pronounce them).

Once Is Not Enough

Product formulations change frequently. Don't assume just because you've used a brand or product in the past it is necessarily safe forever. Don't hesitate to contact the manufacturer if you have questions about ingredients. Most companies are eager to accommodate their gluten-free customers. Call the customer service help line or visit the website.

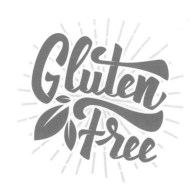

Does a Gluten-Free Label Mean 100% Gluten-Free?

The short answer is not exactly. Experts agree that food can contain a very small amount of gluten and still be tolerated by even those who are sensitive. The trouble is, not everyone agrees on exactly what that tiny amount should be.

The FDA is doing studies and soliciting consumer input on a definition for gluten-free which will eventually govern what appears on labels. For international trade, standards have been set at less than 20 parts per million so that is often the assumed threshold. Meanwhile, there is a private, not-for-profit certification program in place that tests products to see if they contain less than 10 parts per million of gluten. Those that do are allowed to display a "Certified Gluten-Free" logo. Remember, most food is naturally gluten-free. There's no need to look for GF labels on dairy products or a can of beans!

gluten-free nutrition

Is Gluten-Free Healthier?

If you are suffering from celiac disease or gluten intolerance it certainly is! One of the many devastating effects can be the inability of damaged intestines to derive the nutrients your body needs. However, there are steps you should take to ensure you get proper nutrition on a gluten-free diet. Begin by talking to your doctor. Chances are, he or she can suggest a nutritionist you can consult who specializes in gluten free eating.

Gluten-Free Is Not Low-Calorie, Fat-Free or Low-Carb

It is most certainly not a weight-loss regimen. If you simply replace the old white bread, cakes and cookies with gluten-free versions of the same thing, you might be worse off! Most ordinary white flour is fortified to make up for the nutrients lost during processing. Some processed gluten-free flours are nutritionally empty starches. For instance, white rice flour has considerably fewer B vitamins, iron and folate than enriched white flour. It does have more refined carbohydrate, though—not a good trade-off!

On the other hand, going gluten-free can be the start of a healthier diet. You will certainly be paying more attention to the food you eat, which is a huge step in the right direction. Instead of trying to replicate your old diet, start fresh—eat more fresh fruits, vegetables, lean meat and low-fat dairy. If that sounds familiar, it is. It's the basic dietary advice given to everyone, gluten-free or not. Think of your gluten-free lifestyle as an opportunity to try new things, not a life sentence that will deprive you of foods you used to love.

Weighing In on Gluten-Free

Some people gain weight after going gluten-free, some lose. Many newly diagnosed celiac patients are sickly and undernourished because of their disease. Once their bodies begin healing, they regain weight and strength. As gluten-free eating has become mainstream, some people try it hoping to lose weight. As with most popular diets, this is only successful if you are eating fewer calories and replacing empty ones with food that is more nutritious.

the gluten-free kitchen

How to Start Your New Life

Eating gluten-free means the days of ordering a pizza or picking up fried chicken for dinner at the last minute are over. Don't despair! You are about to encounter a whole new world of flavors and good things to eat. Gluten-free cooking isn't difficult—it's just different. The biggest change may be that you need to cook more and use processed foods less.

For those recently diagnosed with celiac disease, setting up the kitchen to avoid cross contamination is an important first step. If you live alone, purge your place of breads, pastas, flours and other no-no's. If you are living with gluten-eating others, you'll need to stake out a gluten-free zone of your own. Clearly mark gluten-free items and make sure everyone understands they are hands-off. Dishes and pots and pans can be shared, because they can be washed between uses.

The biggest culprit in cross-contamination is the common crumb. Crumbs from regular bread find their way onto work surfaces, into condiment jars and toasters. If you will be toasting gluten-free and regular bread, you may want to invest in a second toaster to make your life easier.

Supermarket Savvy

Before you rush off to buy a cupboard full of specialty products, remember that most basic ingredients are naturally gluten-free. You can pick up any sort of fresh produce, meat or fish without worrying. However, certain convenience foods may not be available in gluten-free form, or can be prohibitively expensive. This doesn't mean you can't have your favorite foods anymore. It just means you will be making some adjustments.

Of course, you will want to stock up on certain things so that you're prepared to eat well on your new diet. In the past, a health food store was the only place to buy specialty flours and mixes. Fortunately, today most supermarkets offer just about everything you need. There are also many reliable online sources that are worth checking out.

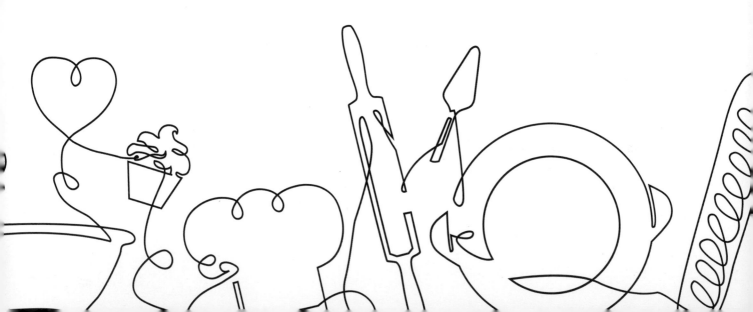

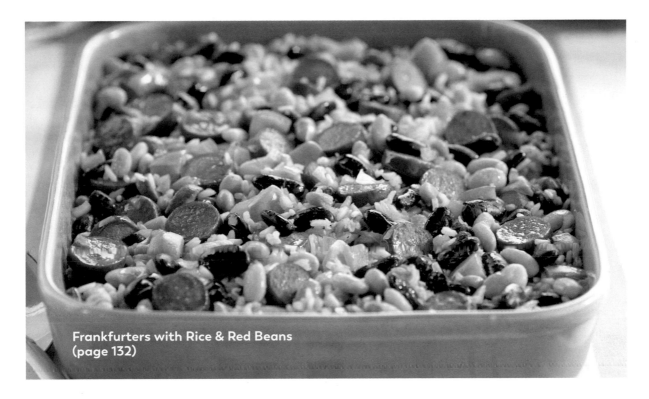

Frankfurters with Rice & Red Beans
(page 132)

cooking gluten-free is easy

There's no need to give away your old cookbooks and recipe cards. Many recipes don't have any problematic ingredients or can easily be converted. When small quantities of flour are needed—for example, to bread chicken or fish—you can substitute any gluten-free flour for regular flour. Stock up on ready-made gluten-free pastas and your old Italian favorites are easy as ever.

Baked goods, especially breads, are a whole lot trickier. While it is certainly possible to buy pre-made gluten-free cookies, cakes and breads, they are expensive and can't compete with homemade treats. Fortunately, it is possible to turn out luscious gluten-free brownies, birthday cakes, pies and even bread with the recipes in this book and a bit of practice. In fact, warm gluten-free bread from your oven is probably tastier and better for you than most supermarket wheat breads!

Flour Power

You won't be surprised to learn that the trick to making gluten-free baked goods is finding a way to replace the power of gluten. In order to replicate the structure and texture it provides, you'll need to combine different nonwheat flours and add xanthan gum. While you can buy premade gluten-free all-purpose flour blends as well as mixes for anything from pancakes to chocolate cake, it's helpful to know a little about the actual flours in them. It seems there are new choices available every day—hemp flour and pea flour are two of the latest. Here are descriptions of some of the more common ones.

flour blends and friends

Why can't there be a single one-for-one substitute for wheat flour? Unfortunately wheat flour performs many different functions and is made up of both protein (the gluten) and starches. It helps make pie crust flaky, cookies chewy and breads crusty. There is no one gluten-free flour that can recreate all those benefits, but that's no reason to give up baking. With two basic flour blends in your refrigerator you can turn out yummy cakes, cookies and even yeast breads.

Gluten-Free All-Purpose Flour Blend
(This blend is for all baked goods not made with yeast.)

- 1 cup white rice flour
- 1 cup sorghum flour
- 1 cup tapioca flour
- 1 cup cornstarch
- 1 cup almond flour or coconut flour

Combine all ingredients in a large bowl. Whisk to make sure the flours are evenly distributed. The recipe can be doubled or tripled. Store in an airtight container in the refrigerator.

When you use this blend, you will need to add ½ teaspoon of xanthan gum for every 1 cup.

Gluten-Free Flour Blend For Breads
(This blend is for recipes that call for yeast.)

- 1 cup brown rice flour
- 1 cup sorghum flour
- ¾ cup millet flour*
- 1 cup tapioca flour
- 1 cup cornstarch
- ⅓ cup instant mashed potato flakes (unflavored)

*If millet flour is not available, chickpea flour may be substituted.

Combine all ingredients in a large bowl. Whisk to make sure flours are evenly distributed. The recipe can be doubled or tripled. Store in an airtight container in the refrigerator.

Blending the Rules

While gluten-free flour blends may seem mysterious at first, they do follow certain logical rules. Basic all-purpose flour blends usually start with 2 parts of grain flour (rice, sorghum or millet), 2 parts of starch (cornstarch or tapioca flour) and 1 part of protein (a bean or nut flour). There are many other considerations. Flavor is one. Nutrition is also important. While a blend made of white rice flour and cornstarch might work, it wouldn't contain much in the way of fiber, protein or vitamins. You can, of course, purchase ready-made blends at the supermarket or on the Internet, but homemade is certainly cheaper and also fresher and better tasting.

Storing and Using Gluten-Free Flour Blends

Most gluten-free flour blends should be stored in the refrigerator or freezer since they contain perishable whole grain or nut flours. Invest in canisters or use clearly marked resealable freezer bags. Bring flours to room temperature before using and remember to rewhisk or shake them so that they are completely combined.

Measuring gluten-free blends is no different than measuring wheat flour, but it is even more important to be accurate. Never pack flour into a measuring cup. Don't dip the measuring cup into the flour, either, since that can compact it. Fluff the flour and spoon it into the cup. Level off the top with the back of a knife.

baking tips and tricks

Gluten-free baking isn't harder, it's just different. The good/bad news is that you'll probably be doing more baking now that you're gluten-free. That's good because you won't be eating all the high-fructose corn syrup and other questionable ingredients in most packaged breads and cookies. The bad news is that you'll have to find the time. There is a bit of a learning curve to gluten-free baking, so don't be discouraged by a failure. Remember, you probably failed at traditional baking a few times, too! Many products that may not look as beautiful as you would like will still taste very good. You can also turn a total failure into gluten-free crumbs to be used another time.

Think Different

Many batters and doughs look drastically different from their gluten-containing counterparts. They tend to be wetter and stickier. Bread dough is more like a thick, stretchy batter. You can celebrate the fact that you'll never need to knead gluten-free bread dough. That's a good thing, since it's so sticky you'd never be able to! You will need to learn to shape sticky dough by using damp hands or a well-oiled spoon or spatula. Parchment paper can be a real help for lining pans and transporting soft doughs.

You will be using xanthan gum to provide elasticity and hold doughs together. It's important to measure it very carefully. Too much and your baked goods will shrink after baking. You may find a dense, gummy layer of dough near the bottom of the pan.

Smarty Pans

Pans are a critical part of the recipe. Black or dark metal pans can be a problem because they absorb heat more quickly. The recipes in this book were tested in pans and on baking sheets with light, shiny surfaces. If you must use dark pans, try lining them with foil, watch carefully and lower oven temperatures or cooking times if necessary. Disposable aluminum pans work surprisingly well for many recipes.

Pan size can be the difference between a perfect cake or loaf and a flop—literally! The same batter intended for a 9×5-inch loaf pan, can puff up over the top of an 8×4-inch pan and then collapse. Measure pan size across the top from inside edge to inside edge.

Temperamental Temperatures

Oven temperatures are also important. If you don't have an oven thermometer, you may want to get one. Home ovens are frequently off by as much as 50 degrees. While you're at it, pick up an inexpensive instant-read thermometer, too. It's a big help in knowing when bread is done (190° to 200°F). Gluten-free goods tend to brown more quickly. They can look done on the outside when they're still gooey in the center so be ready to cover things with a sheet of foil to prevent burning.

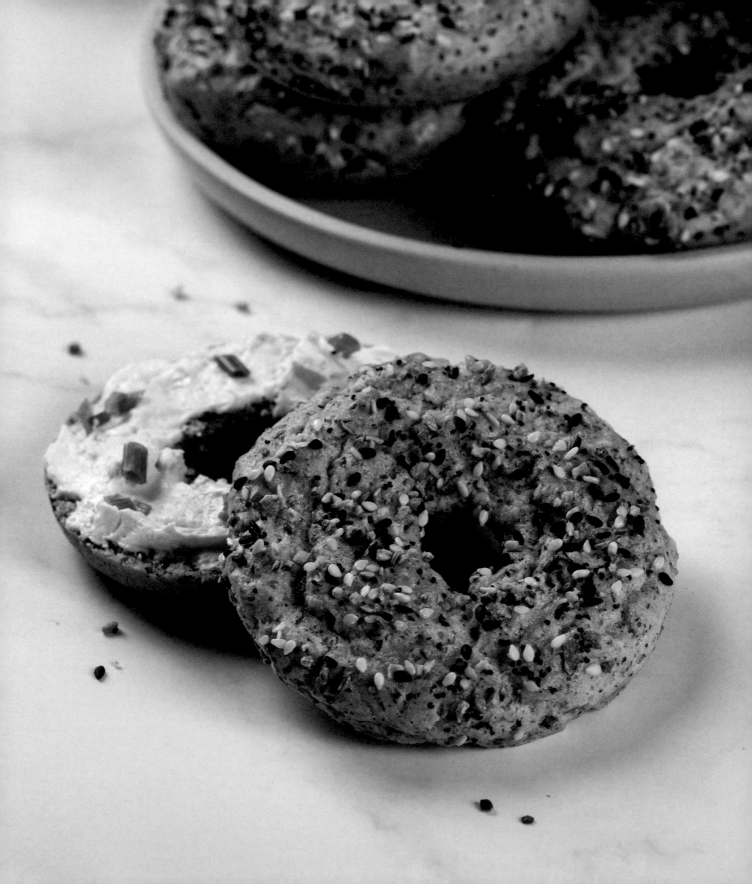

morning meals

Everything Bagels
Makes 12 bagels

6   eggs at room temperature, separated

¼   teaspoon cream of tartar

2   cups almond flour

3½ teaspoons baking powder

½   teaspoon salt

¼   teaspoon garlic powder

6   tablespoons butter, melted and cooled slightly

½   cup finely shredded Asiago cheese

2   tablespoons everything bagel seasoning

1. Preheat oven to 350°F. Spray 12 cavities of doughnut pans with nonstick cooking spray.

2. Place egg whites and cream of tartar in large bowl; attach whisk attachment to stand mixer. Whip egg whites on high speed 2 minutes or until stiff peaks form. Transfer egg whites to medium bowl.

3. Combine almond flour, baking powder, salt and garlic powder in mixer bowl. Add melted butter and egg yolks; mix on medium speed until well blended. Add cheese; mix well.

4. Stir one third of egg whites into almond flour mixture with spatula until well blended. Gently fold in remaining egg whites until thoroughly blended. Scoop mixture into large resealable food storage bag; cut off one corner. Pipe about ¼ cup batter into each doughnut cavity. Sprinkle each with ½ teaspoon everything bagel seasoning.

5. Bake about 10 minutes or until bagels are golden brown and set. Cool in pans 2 minutes. Remove to wire rack; serve warm or cool completely.

Everything Bagel Muffins: If you don't have doughnut pans or would prefer to make muffins instead, scoop batter into 12 greased standard muffin pan cups. Sprinkle with bagel seasoning. Bake 15 minutes or until tops are golden brown and toothpick inserted into centers comes out clean.

Crustless Ham & Spinach Tart

Makes 4 servings

1 teaspoon olive oil

1 cup finely chopped onion

2 cloves garlic, minced

1 package (10 ounces) frozen chopped spinach, thawed and squeezed dry

3 slices deli ham, cut into strips (3 ounces total)

1 cup milk

3 eggs

¼ cup plus 2 tablespoons grated Parmesan cheese, divided

1 tablespoon minced fresh basil *or* 2 teaspoons dried basil

½ teaspoon black pepper

⅛ teaspoon ground nutmeg

1. Preheat oven to 350°F. Spray 9-inch glass pie plate with nonstick cooking spray.

2. Heat oil in medium skillet over medium-high heat. Add onion; cook and stir 2 minutes or until softened. Add garlic; cook and stir 1 minute. Stir in spinach and ham. Spread mixture evenly in prepared pie plate.

3. Whisk milk, eggs, ¼ cup cheese, basil, pepper and nutmeg in medium bowl until well blended. Pour mixture over spinach mixture.

4. Bake 50 minutes or until knife inserted into center comes out clean. Sprinkle with remaining 2 tablespoons cheese. Cut into wedges to serve.

Tip: Leftover tart wedges make great grab-and-go breakfasts. Eat them cold or heat them up in the microwave.

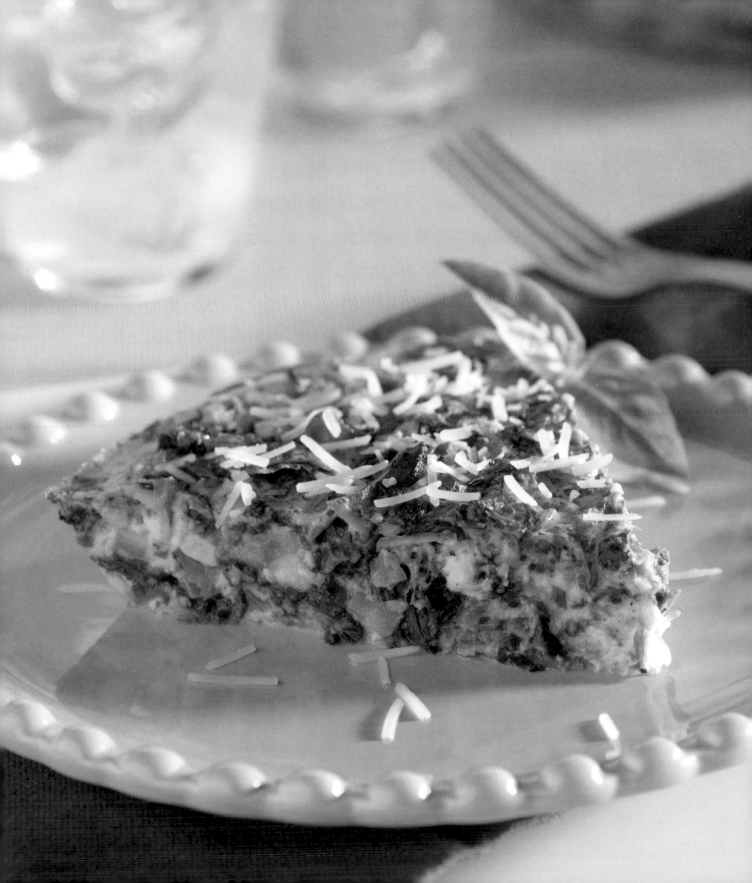

Classic Waffles

Makes 5 (6-inch) waffles

2 eggs

½ cup plain yogurt

½ cup whole milk

1 cup one-to-one gluten-free baking flour*

1 tablespoon sugar

1 teaspoon baking powder

1 teaspoon baking soda

½ teaspoon salt

2 tablespoons butter, melted

Maple syrup and additional butter

Or use any gluten-free all-purpose flour blend that contains xanthan gum, or make your own with the recipe on page 12.

1. Preheat waffle iron according to manufacturer's directions.

2. Beat eggs in large bowl until light and fluffy. Whisk in yogurt and milk.

3. Combine flour, sugar, baking powder, baking soda and salt in medium bowl. Gradually whisk yogurt mixture into flour mixture until smooth. Whisk in melted butter.

4. Add batter to waffle iron by ½ cupfuls for 6-inch waffles (or adjust amount depending on waffle iron); cook until steaming stops and waffles are crisp and browned. Serve with maple syrup and additional butter.

Note: Refrigerate or freeze leftover waffles; reheat in toaster oven until crisp.

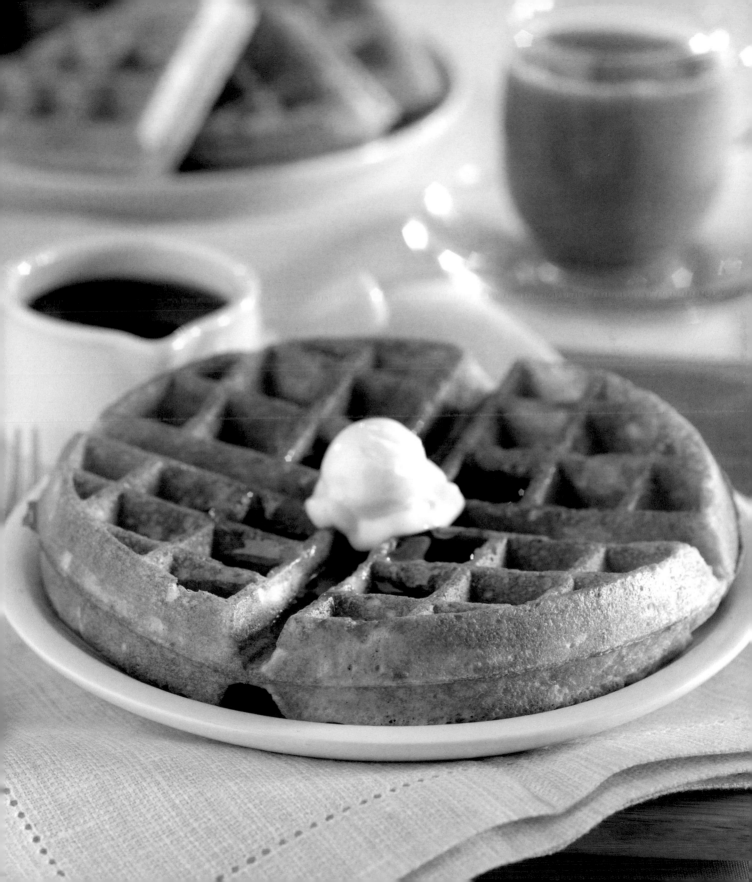

Bacon & Cheese Grits

Makes 4 servings

- **4** thick-cut slices bacon, chopped
- **2** cups milk
- **½** cup quick-cooking grits
- **1½** cups (6 ounces) shredded sharp Cheddar cheese *or* 6 slices American cheese, torn into bite-size pieces
- **2** tablespoons butter
- **1** teaspoon Worcestershire sauce
- **½** teaspoon salt
- **⅛** teaspoon ground red pepper (optional)

1. Heat medium skillet over medium heat. Add bacon; cook and stir until crisp. Remove bacon with slotted spoon; drain on paper towel-lined plate.

2. Meanwhile, bring milk to a boil in large saucepan over medium-high heat. Slowly stir in grits; return to a boil. Reduce heat to low; cover and simmer 5 minutes, stirring frequently.

3. Remove from heat; stir in cheese, butter, Worcestershire sauce, salt and ground red pepper, if desired. Cover; let stand 2 minutes or until cheese is melted. Scoop into bowls; top with bacon.

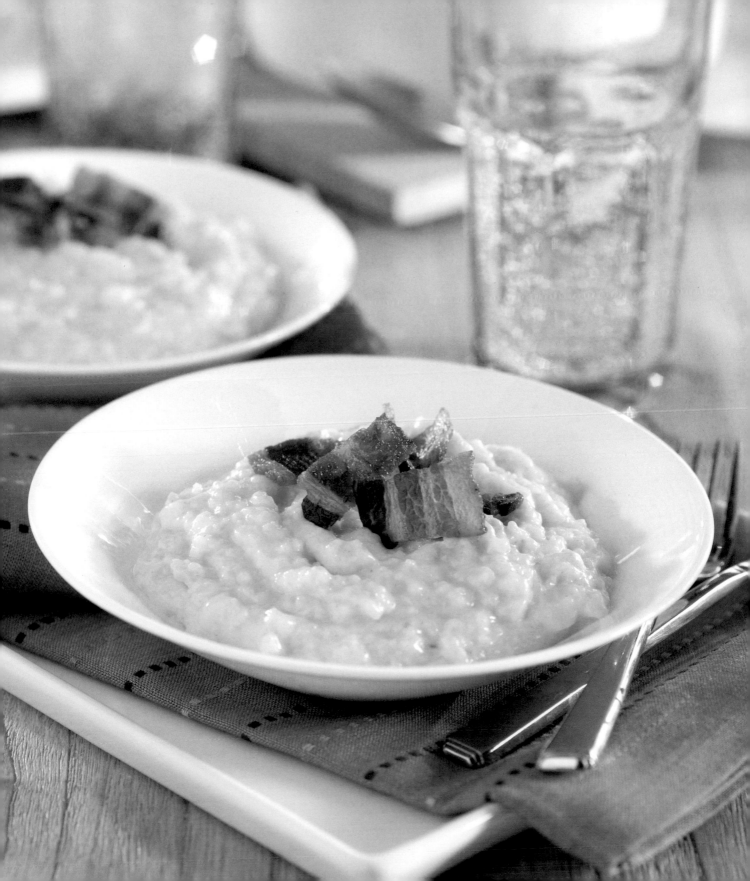

Banana Split Breakfast Bowl

Makes 4 servings

2½ tablespoons sliced almonds

2½ tablespoons chopped walnuts

3 cups vanilla yogurt

1⅓ cups sliced fresh strawberries
     (about 12 medium)

2 bananas

½ cup drained pineapple tidbits

1. Combine almonds and walnuts in small skillet; cook and stir over medium heat 2 minutes or until lightly browned. Immediately remove from skillet; cool completely.

2. Spoon yogurt into serving bowl. Layer with strawberries, bananas and pineapple; sprinkle with toasted almonds and walnuts.

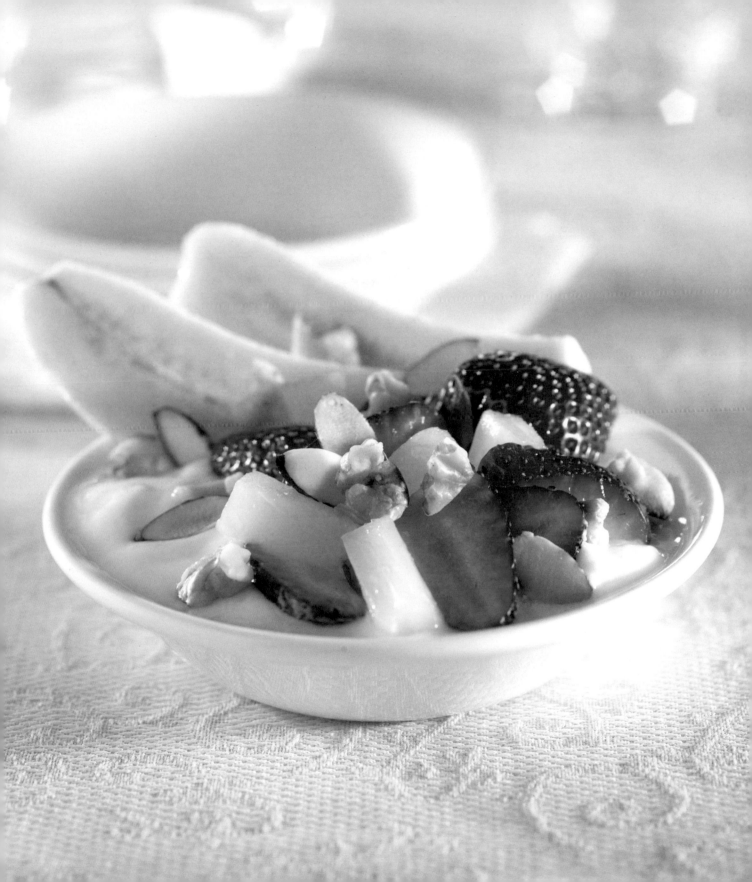

Buttermilk Pancakes

Makes 16 (4-inch) pancakes

2 cups one-to-one gluten-free baking flour*

1½ tablespoons sugar

1 teaspoon baking powder

1 teaspoon baking soda

½ teaspoon salt

2¼ cups buttermilk

2 eggs

2 tablespoons butter, melted and cooled

Vegetable oil

Maple syrup and additional butter

Or use any gluten-free all-purpose flour blend that contains xanthan gum, or make your own with the recipe on page 12.

1. Whisk flour, sugar, baking powder, baking soda and salt in large bowl. Whisk buttermilk, eggs and 2 tablespoons butter in small bowl. Gradually whisk buttermilk mixture into flour mixture until smooth.

2. Heat oil on griddle or in large nonstick skillet over medium heat. Pour ¼ cupfuls of batter 2 inches apart onto griddle. Cook 2 minutes or until lightly browned and edges begin to bubble. Turn over; cook 2 minutes or until lightly browned. Repeat with remaining batter. Serve pancakes with maple syrup and additional butter.

Note: If you do not plan on serving the pancakes right away, keep them warm in a 200°F oven.

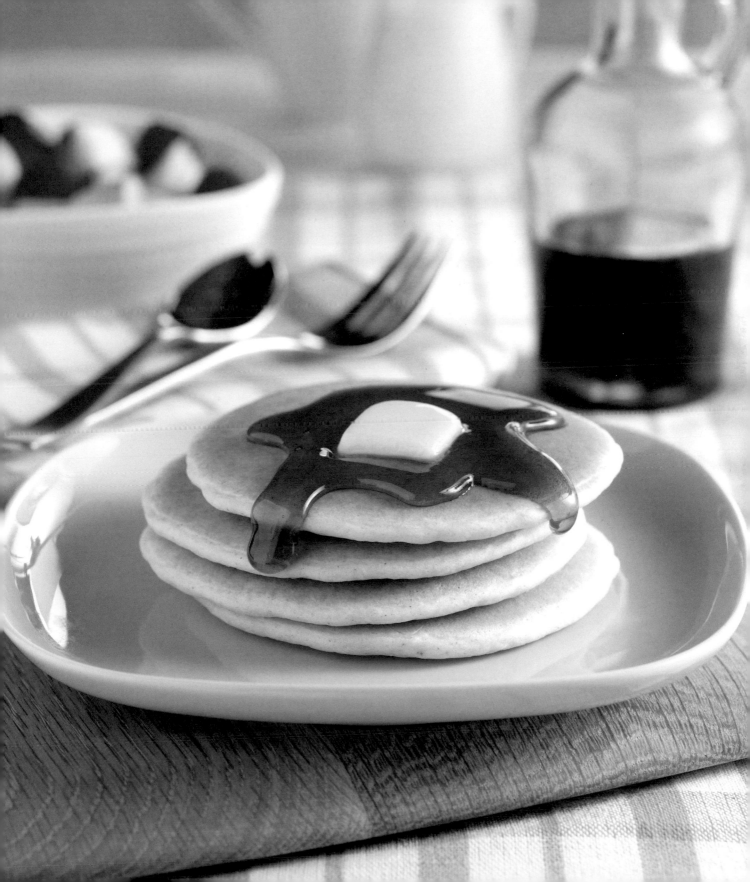

Almond Flour Pound Cake

Makes 9 to 12 slices

2 cups almond flour

1 teaspoon baking powder

1 teaspoon salt

¼ teaspoon ground ginger

¼ teaspoon ground cardamom

½ cup (1 stick) butter, softened

4 ounces cream cheese, softened

¾ cup granulated sugar

2 tablespoons packed brown sugar

4 eggs

1 teaspoon vanilla

1 tablespoon sliced almonds

1. Preheat oven to 350°F. Spray 9×5-inch loaf pan with nonstick cooking spray or line with parchment paper.

2. Combine almond flour, baking powder, salt, ginger and cardamom in medium bowl.

3. Beat butter, cream cheese, granulated sugar and brown sugar in large bowl with electric mixer at medium speed until well blended. Add eggs, one at a time, beating well after each addition, followed by vanilla. Gradually add dry ingredients, beating until blended. Pour batter into prepared pan; sprinkle with sliced almonds.

4. Bake 45 to 55 minutes or until toothpick inserted into center comes out clean. Cool in pan on wire rack 10 minutes. Remove from pan; cool completely. Store leftovers in the refrigerator.

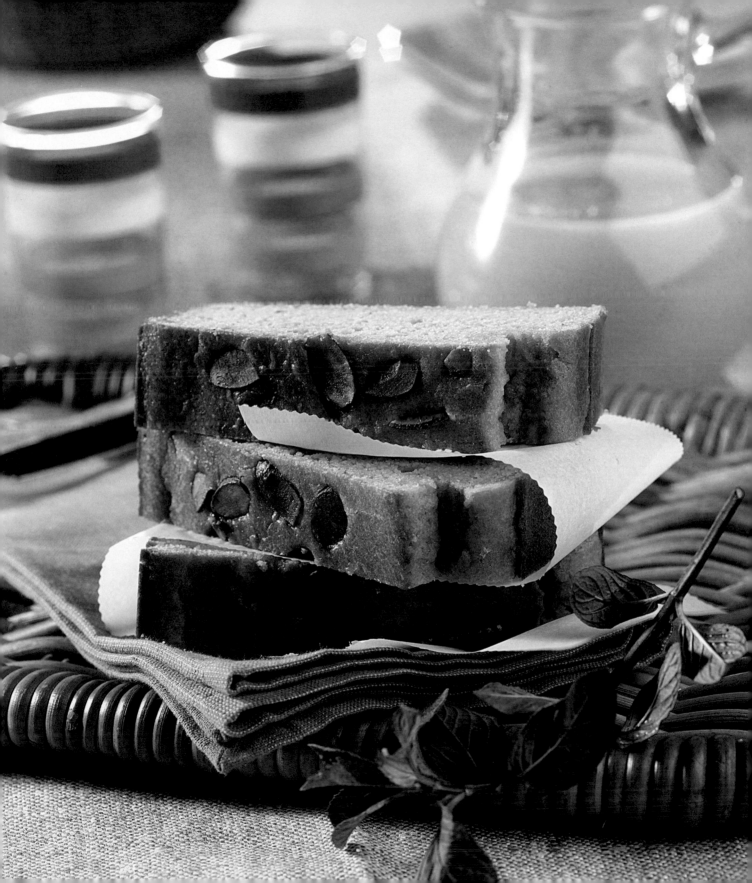

Roasted Tomato Quiche

Makes 6 servings

1 pint grape tomatoes

1 tablespoon olive oil

Salt and black pepper

2½ cups riced cauliflower (fresh or frozen)

½ cup shredded Parmesan cheese

6 eggs, divided

¾ teaspoon salt, divided

½ teaspoon black pepper, divided

¾ cup milk

½ cup (2 ounces) shredded mozzarella cheese

2 cloves garlic, minced

½ teaspoon chopped fresh thyme

1. Preheat oven to 350°F. Place tomatoes in shallow baking dish; drizzle with oil and sprinkle lightly with salt and pepper. Bake 1 hour, stirring once or twice.*

2. *Increase oven temperature to 425°F.* Spray 9-inch pie plate with nonstick cooking spray.

3. Place cauliflower in large microwavable bowl; cover with plastic wrap and cut slit to vent. Microwave on HIGH 4 minutes; stir. Cover and cook on HIGH 4 minutes. Remove cover; cool slightly. Place cauliflower on double layer of paper towels; fold over paper towels and squeeze to remove excess moisture. Return to bowl. Add Parmesan cheese, 1 egg, ½ teaspoon salt and ¼ teaspoon pepper; mix well. Press onto bottom and up side of prepared pie plate. Bake crust 15 minutes. Remove from oven; place on sheet pan.

4. *Reduce oven temperature to 375°F.* Whisk remaining 5 eggs, milk, mozzarella cheese, garlic, thyme, remaining ¼ teaspoon salt and ¼ teaspoon pepper in medium bowl until well blended. Place tomatoes in crust; pour egg mixture over tomatoes. Bake 45 minutes or until thin knife inserted into center comes out clean (a little cheese is okay). Cool 10 minutes before slicing.

*Tomatoes can be roasted a day or two in advance. Store them in an airtight container in the refrigerator until ready to use.

Note: To make riced cauliflower, cut one head of cauliflower into 1-inch florets. Working in batches, place cauliflower in bowl of food processor and pulse the florets until they form small rice-size pieces. If there are any large chunks left behind, pick them out and add them to your next batch. Or grate a whole head of cauliflower on the large holes of a box grater into a large bowl, rotating until all the florets are shredded.

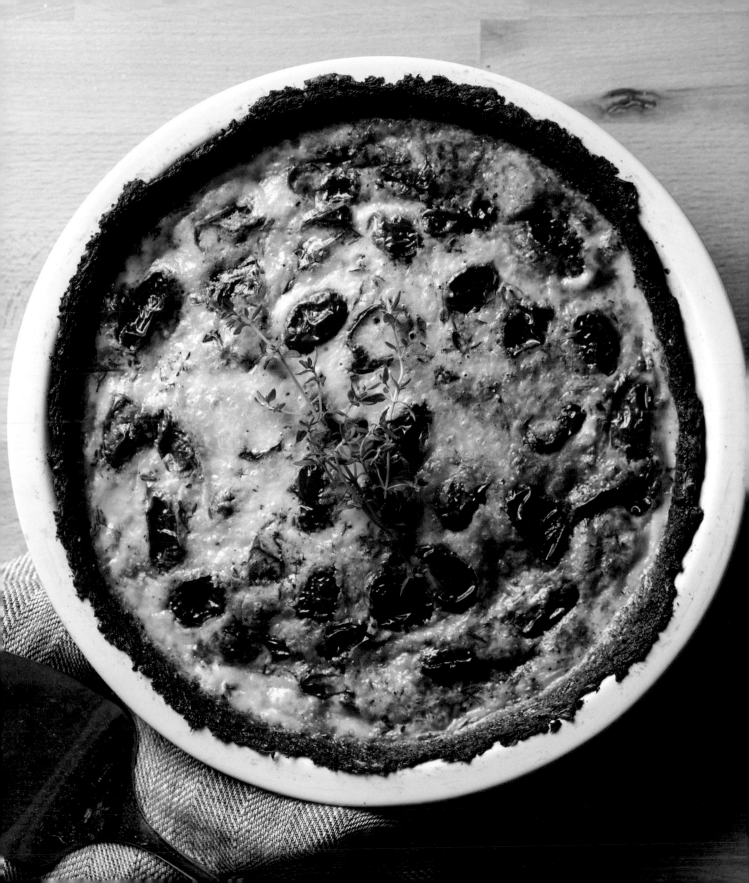

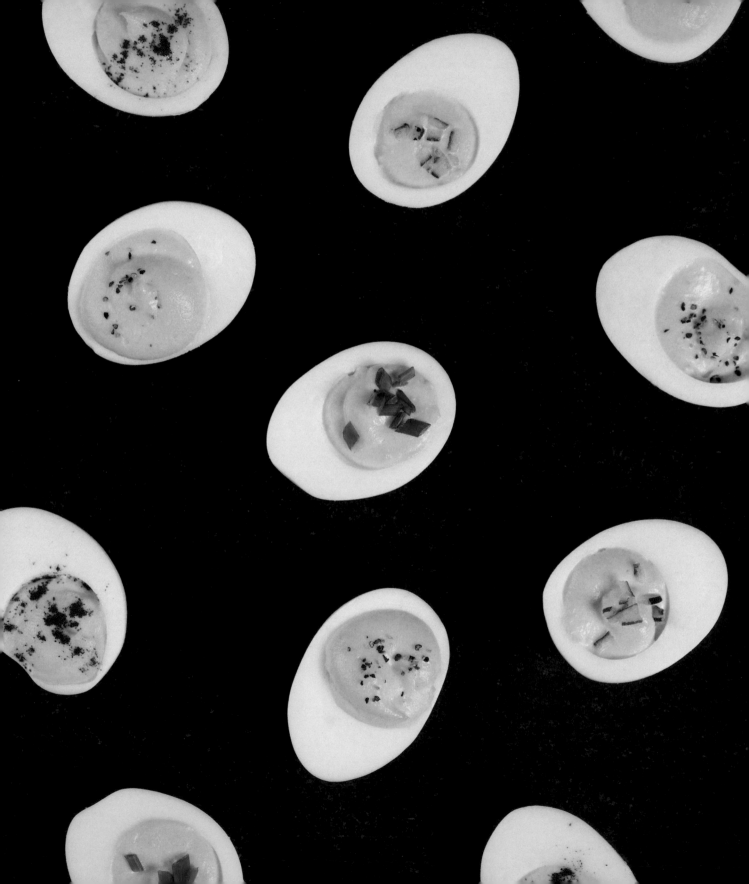

snacks *and* appetizers

Classic Deviled Eggs
Makes 12 deviled eggs

6 eggs

3 tablespoons mayonnaise

½ teaspoon cider vinegar

½ teaspoon yellow mustard

⅛ teaspoon salt

Optional toppings: black pepper, paprika, minced fresh chives and/or minced red onion (optional)

1. Bring medium saucepan of water to a boil. Gently add eggs with slotted spoon. Reduce heat to maintain a simmer; cook 12 minutes. Meanwhile, fill medium bowl with cold water and ice cubes. Drain eggs and place in ice water; cool 10 minutes.

2. Carefully peel eggs. Cut eggs in half; place yolks in small bowl. Add mayonnaise, vinegar, mustard and salt; mash until well blended. Spoon mixture into egg whites; garnish with desired toppings.

Sweet & Spicy Popcorn Clusters

Makes 6 servings

½ cup sugar

6 tablespoons (¾ stick) butter

4 teaspoons light corn syrup

½ teaspoon salt

½ teaspoon ground red pepper

12 cups popped popcorn (oil-popped, air-popped or butter-flavor microwave popcorn)

1. Combine sugar, butter, corn syrup, salt and ground red pepper in large saucepan. Bring to a boil over medium heat; boil 3 minutes. Remove from heat.

2. Immediately stir in popcorn; toss to coat evenly.

3. Spread mixture in single layer on baking sheets. Let stand 1 hour to cool completely. Break into clusters. Store in airtight container.

Tip: For oil-popped popcorn, heat ¼ cup vegetable oil in large 6-quart saucepan over medium-high heat; add 4 unpopped popcorn kernels and cover saucepan with tight-fitting lid. When popcorn pops, add ½ cup popcorn kernels. Cover tightly with lid and cook 2 to 3 minutes or until popcorn slows to about 1 second between pops, carefully shaking pan occasionally.

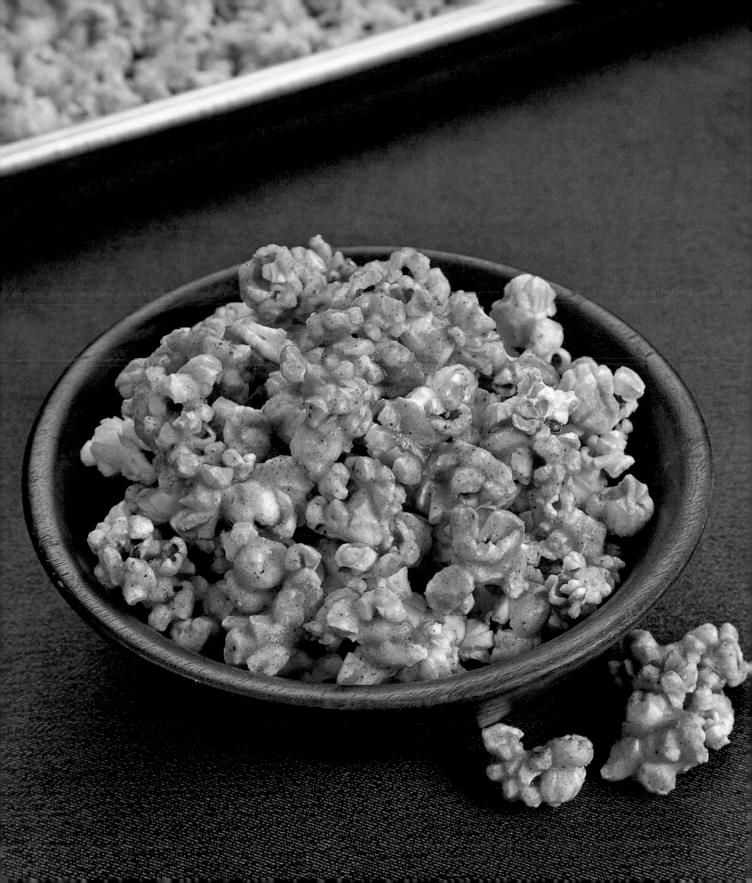

Cheddar Crackers

Makes 24 crackers

1½ cups brown rice flour

1 teaspoon garlic powder

1 teaspoon Italian seasoning

½ teaspoon salt

½ cup (2 ounces) finely grated
   sharp Cheddar cheese

6 tablespoons (¾ stick) cold
   butter, cut into ½-inch cubes

½ cup cold water

1. Combine brown rice flour, garlic powder, Italian seasoning and salt in food processor; process until well blended. Add cheese and butter; pulse until coarse crumbs form. Add water; process until dough forms.

2. Divide dough into two pieces; wrap in plastic wrap and refrigerate 20 minutes.

3. Preheat oven to 350°F. Line baking sheets with parchment paper.

4. Place each dough half between two pieces of parchment paper; roll out to ⅟₁₆-inch thickness. Refrigerate 5 minutes.

5. Cut dough into 2½-inch squares; place on prepared baking sheets.

6. Bake 15 minutes or until crackers are golden and crisp, rotating baking sheets after 10 minutes. Cool on baking sheets 10 minutes. Remove to wire racks; cool completely.

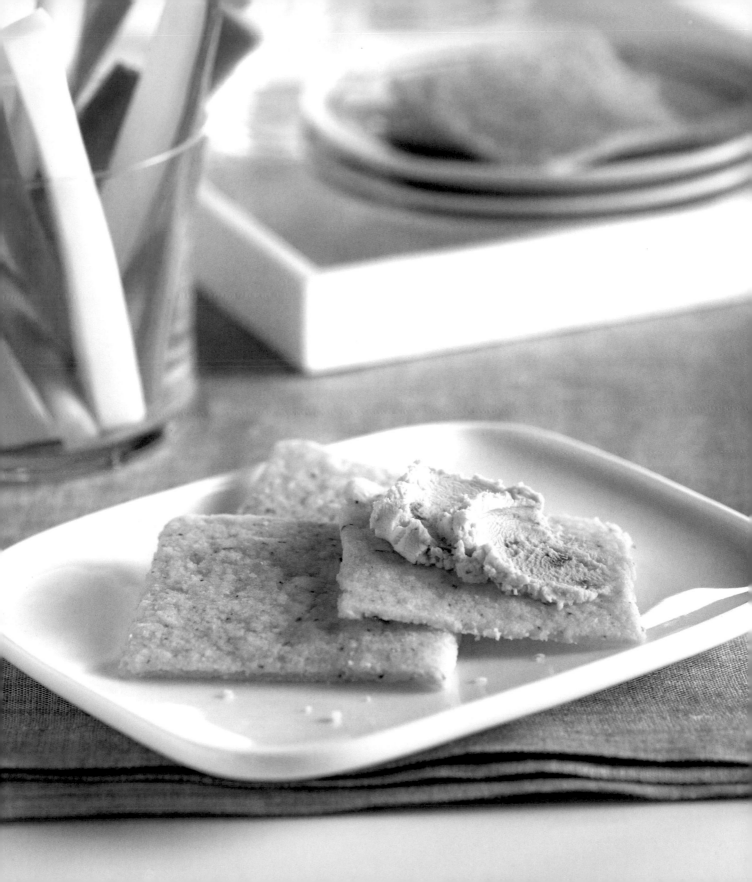

Asparagus Roll-Ups

Makes 24 roll-ups

24 asparagus spears, tough ends trimmed (about 1 pound)

1 teaspoon salt

4 ounces cream cheese, softened

24 thin salami slices (about 8 ounces)

1. Cut asparagus into lengths 1 inch longer than width of salami. Reserve bottoms for another use. Place about ½ inch of water in large skillet; add salt. Bring to a simmer over medium heat. Add asparagus; simmer 4 minutes or until crisp-tender. Drain and immediately immerse in cold water to stop cooking. Drain and pat dry with paper towel.

2. Spread about 1 teaspoon cream cheese evenly over one side of each salami slice. Roll up 1 asparagus spear in each salami slice.

3. Serve immediately or cover and refrigerate until ready to serve; let stand at room temperature 10 minutes before serving.

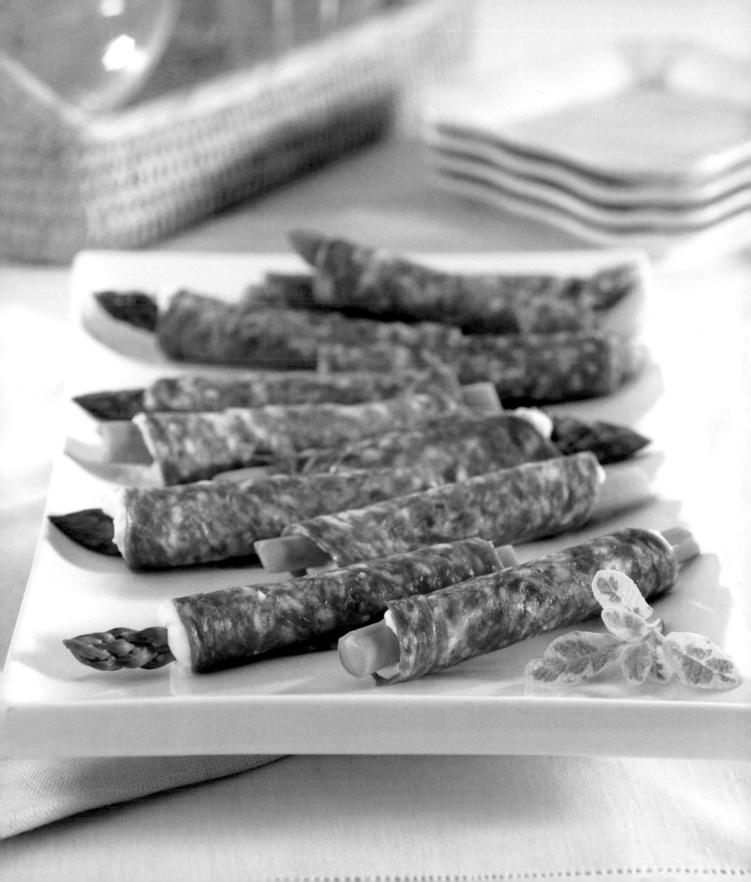

Power-Packed Snack Bars

Makes 16 bars

3 cups puffed millet cereal

1 cup dried fruit bits

¼ cup roasted sunflower kernels

1 teaspoon ground cinnamon

½ cup creamy peanut, almond or soynut butter

½ cup honey

2 tablespoons packed brown sugar

1. Line 8- to 9-inch square baking pan with parchment paper. Spray with nonstick cooking spray.

2. Combine millet, dried fruit, sunflower kernels and cinnamon in large bowl; mix well.

3. Combine peanut butter, honey and brown sugar in medium microwavable bowl. Microwave on HIGH 15 seconds or until melted and smooth. Stir into millet mixture until well combined and evenly coated.

4. Pour mixture into prepared pan; press firmly into even layer. Cover and refrigerate at least 2 hours or until firm. Cut into bars.

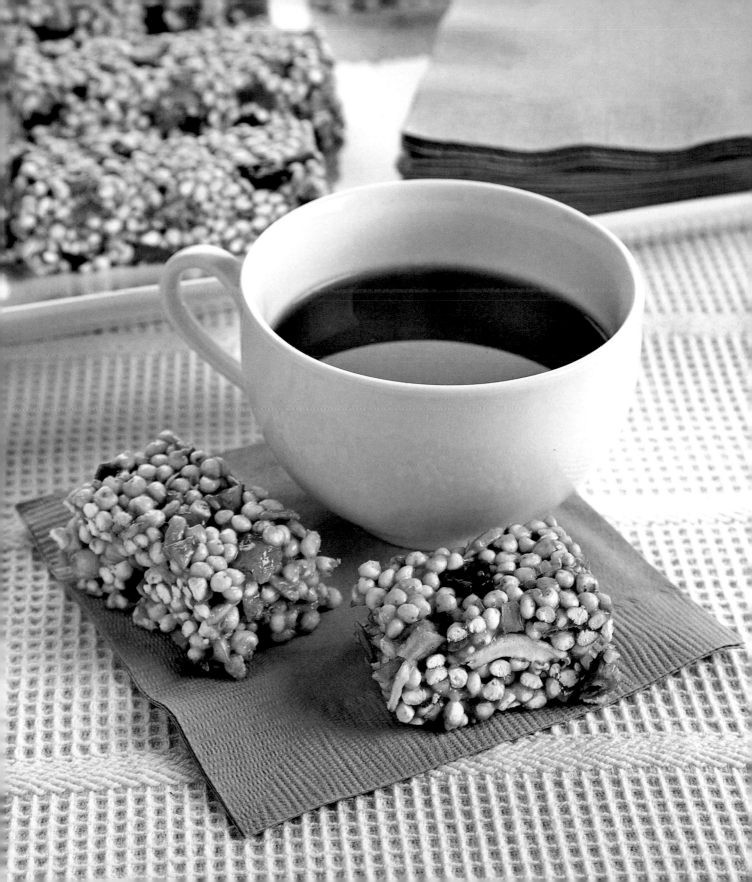

Smoked Salmon Spread

Makes 12 servings (1½ cups)

1 package (8 ounces) cream cheese, softened

3 ounces smoked salmon (lox), coarsely chopped

2 tablespoons fresh lemon juice

1 tablespoon chopped fresh dill

1 tablespoon capers

Cut-up fresh vegetables and/or gluten-free crackers

1. Combine cream cheese, salmon, lemon juice, dill and capers in small bowl; mix well.

2. Serve immediately or cover and refrigerate until ready to serve. Serve with vegetables and/or crackers.

Tip: Try this spread with Everything Bagels (page 15) for breakfast or a quick packable lunch. This spread can be prepared up to 3 days in advance and stored, tightly covered, in the refrigerator.

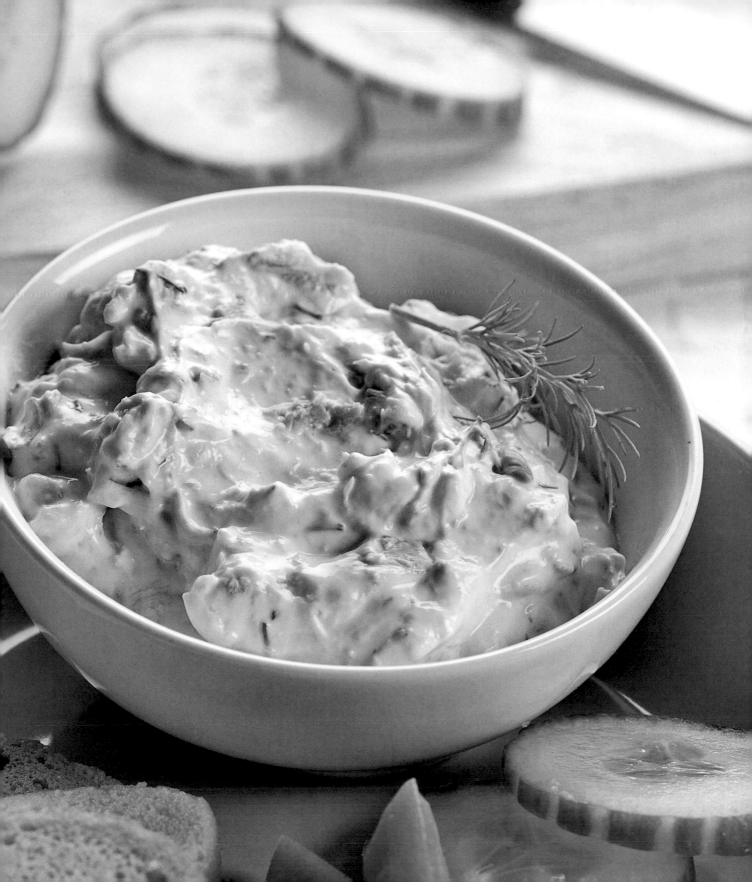

Sweet Hot Chicken Wings

Makes about 36 wings

3 pounds chicken wings

¾ cup salsa

⅔ cup honey

⅓ cup tamari or gluten-free soy sauce

¼ cup Dijon mustard

2 tablespoons vegetable oil

1 tablespoon grated fresh ginger

½ teaspoon grated orange peel

½ teaspoon grated lemon peel

Ranch dressing (optional)

1. Cut off and discard wing tips from chicken. Cut each wing in half at joint. Place wings in 13×9-inch baking dish.

2. Combine salsa, honey, soy sauce, mustard, oil, ginger, orange peel and lemon peel in small bowl; mix well. Pour over wings. Cover and marinate in refrigerator at least 6 hours or overnight.

3. Preheat oven to 400°F. Line large baking sheet with foil. Place wings in single layer on prepared baking sheet. Pour marinade evenly over wings.

4. Bake 40 to 45 minutes until wings are browned and cooked through. Serve warm with ranch dressing, if desired.

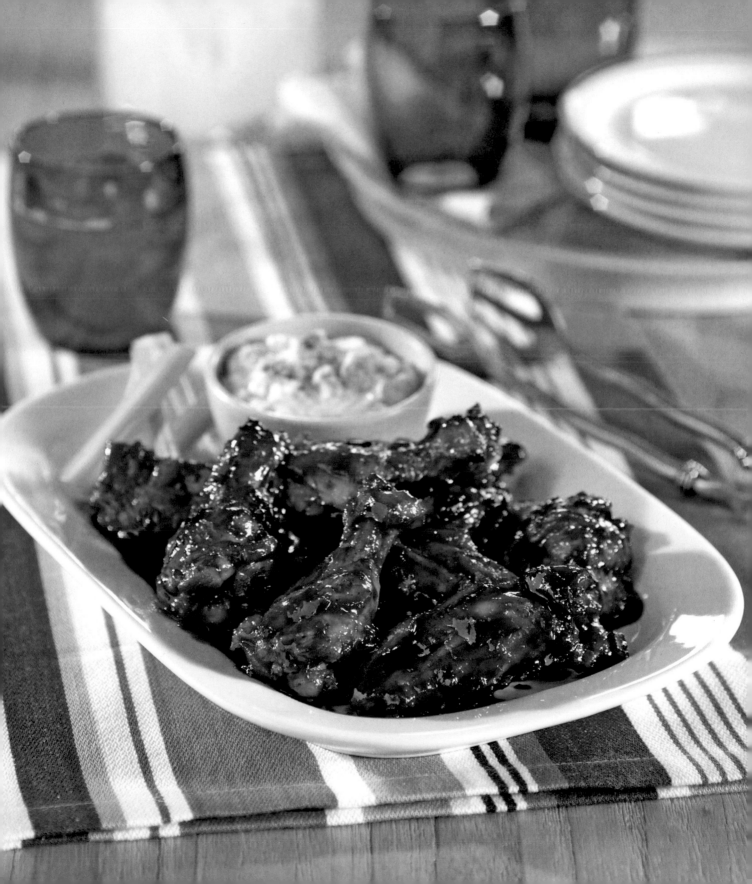

Crispy Oven Fries with Herbed Dipping Sauce

Makes 3 servings

Herbed Dipping Sauce (recipe follows)

2 large unpeeled baking potatoes

2 tablespoons vegetable oil

1 teaspoon kosher salt

1. Preheat oven to 425°F. Line two baking sheets with foil; spray with nonstick cooking spray. Prepare Herbed Dipping Sauce.

2. Cut potatoes lengthwise into ¼-inch slices, then cut each slice into ¼-inch strips. Combine potato strips and oil in large bowl; spread on prepared baking sheets in single layer.

3. Bake 25 minutes. Turn fries over; bake 15 minutes or until light golden brown and crisp. Sprinkle with salt. Serve immediately with Herbed Dipping Sauce.

Herbed Dipping Sauce: Stir ½ cup mayonnaise, 2 tablespoons chopped fresh herbs (such as basil, parsley, oregano and/or dill), 1 teaspoon salt and ½ teaspoon black pepper in small bowl until smooth and well blended. Cover; refrigerate until ready to serve.

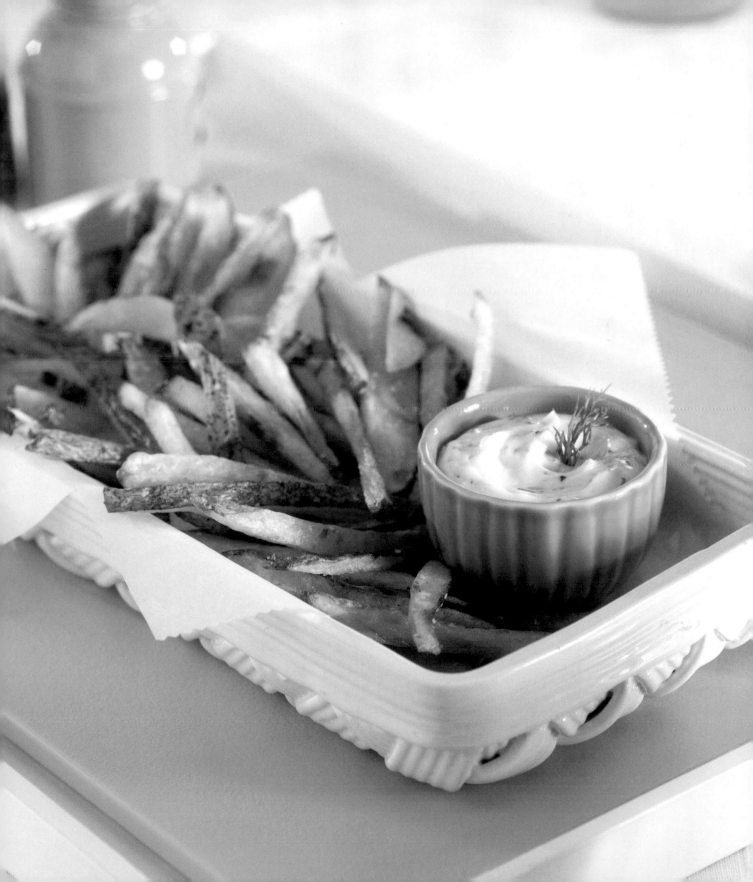

Sweet & Savory Onion Dip

Makes 3 cups dip (about 24 servings)

1 tablespoon olive oil

3 onions, diced

1 teaspoon salt

2 cups plain Greek yogurt

¼ cup grated Parmesan cheese

2 tablespoons fresh lemon juice

⅛ teaspoon ground red pepper

Cut-up fresh vegetables and/or potato chips

1. Heat oil in large nonstick skillet over medium-high heat. Add onions; cook and stir 6 to 8 minutes or until softened. Stir in salt. Reduce heat to low; cook 15 minutes or until onions are deep golden brown; stirring occasionally.

2. Stir yogurt, cheese, lemon juice,and ground red pepper in large bowl until smooth and well blended.

3. Stir onions into yogurt mixture. Cover and refrigerate at least 2 hours before serving. Serve with vegetables and/or chips for dipping.

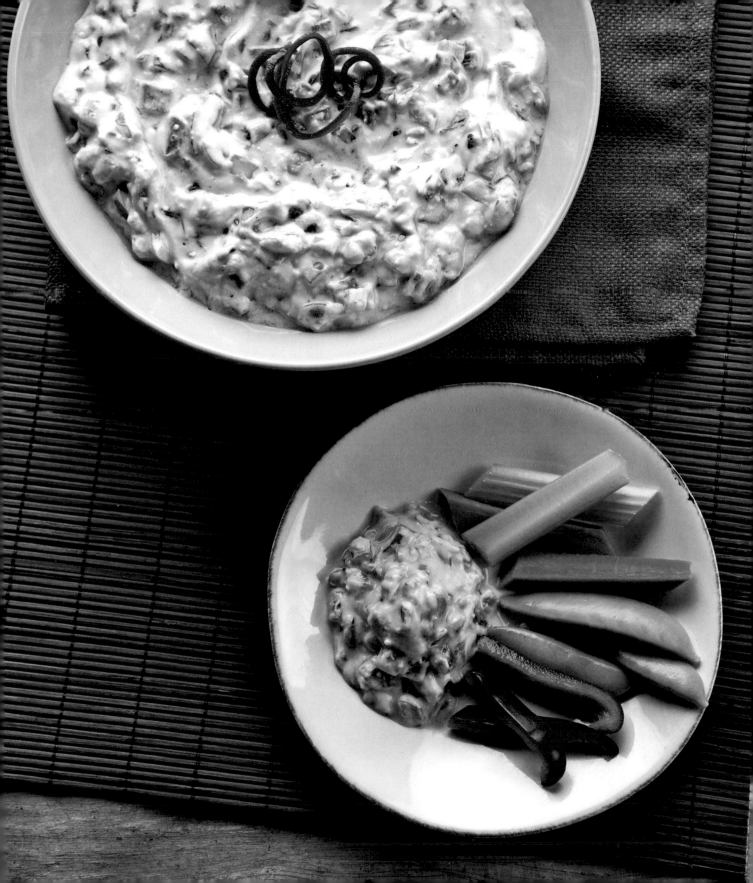

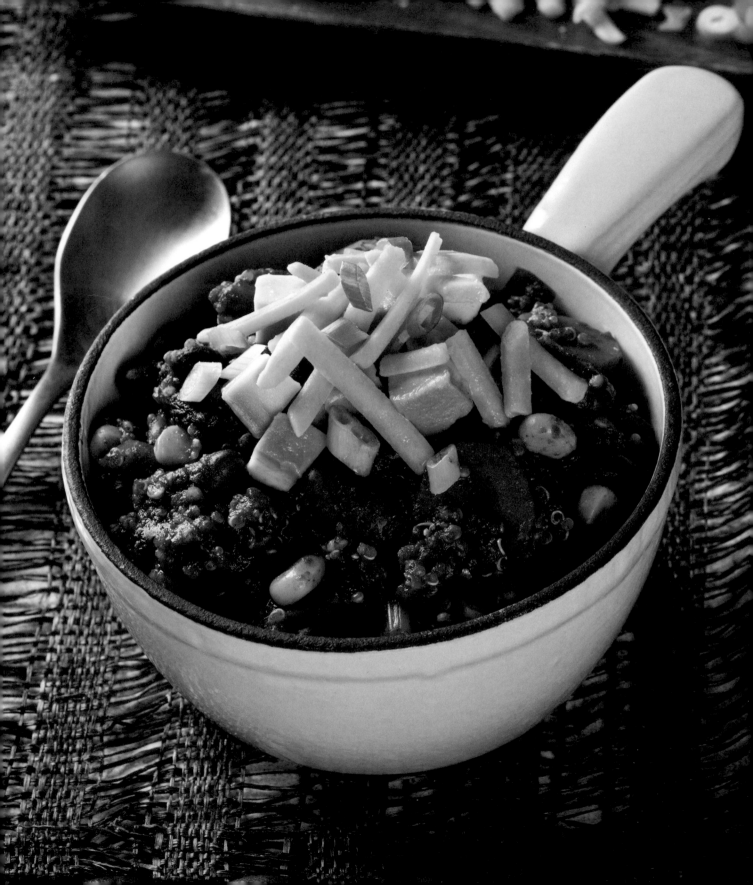

soups *and* salads

Vegetarian Quinoa Chili

Makes 6 servings

2   tablespoons vegetable oil

1   large onion, chopped

1   red bell pepper, chopped

1   large carrot, diced

1   stalk celery, diced

1   jalapeño pepper, seeded and finely chopped

1   tablespoon minced garlic

1   tablespoon chili powder

2   teaspoons ground cumin

1   teaspoon salt

1   can (28 ounces) crushed tomatoes

1   can (about 15 ounces) kidney beans, rinsed and drained

1   cup water

1   cup fresh or frozen corn

½   cup uncooked quinoa, rinsed well in fine-mesh strainer

Optional toppings: diced avocado, shredded Cheddar cheese and/or sliced green onions

1. Heat oil in large saucepan over medium-high heat. Add onion, bell pepper, carrot and celery; cook 10 minutes or until vegetables are softened, stirring occasionally. Add jalapeño, garlic, chili powder, cumin and salt; cook 1 minute or until fragrant.

2. Add tomatoes, beans, water, corn and quinoa; bring to a boil. Reduce heat to low; cover and simmer 1 hour, stirring occasionally.

3. Spoon into bowls; serve with desired toppings.

Entrée Chopped Salad

Makes 8 to 10 servings (20 cups)

Dressing

1½ teaspoons salt

1½ teaspoons dried oregano

¾ teaspoon sugar

¾ teaspoon onion powder

¾ teaspoon dried parsley flakes

½ teaspoon garlic powder

¼ teaspoon dried basil

¼ teaspoon black pepper

⅛ teaspoon dried thyme

⅛ teaspoon celery salt

⅓ cup white balsamic vinegar

¼ cup Dijon mustard

⅔ cup extra virgin olive oil

Salad

1 head iceberg lettuce, chopped

1 head romaine lettuce, chopped

1 can (about 14 ounces) hearts of palm or artichoke hearts, quartered lengthwise then sliced crosswise

1 large avocado, diced

1½ cups crumbled blue cheese

2 hard-cooked eggs, chopped (see Tip)

1 ripe tomato, chopped

½ small red onion, finely chopped

12 slices bacon, crisp-cooked and crumbled

1. For dressing, combine salt, oregano, sugar, onion powder, parsley flakes, garlic powder, basil, pepper, thyme and celery salt in medium bowl. Whisk in vinegar and mustard. Gradually whisk in oil in thin steady stream until well blended. Set aside until ready to use. (Dressing can be made up to 1 week in advance; refrigerate in jar with tight-fitting lid.)

2. For salad, combine iceberg lettuce, romaine lettuce, hearts of palm, avocado, cheese, eggs, tomato, onion and bacon in large bowl. Add dressing; toss to coat.

Tip: For hard-cooked eggs, bring medium saucepan of water to a boil. Gently add eggs with slotted spoon. Reduce heat to maintain a simmer; cook 12 minutes. Meanwhile, fill medium bowl with cold water and ice cubes. Drain eggs and place in ice water; cool 10 minutes. Peel when eggs are cool enough to handle.

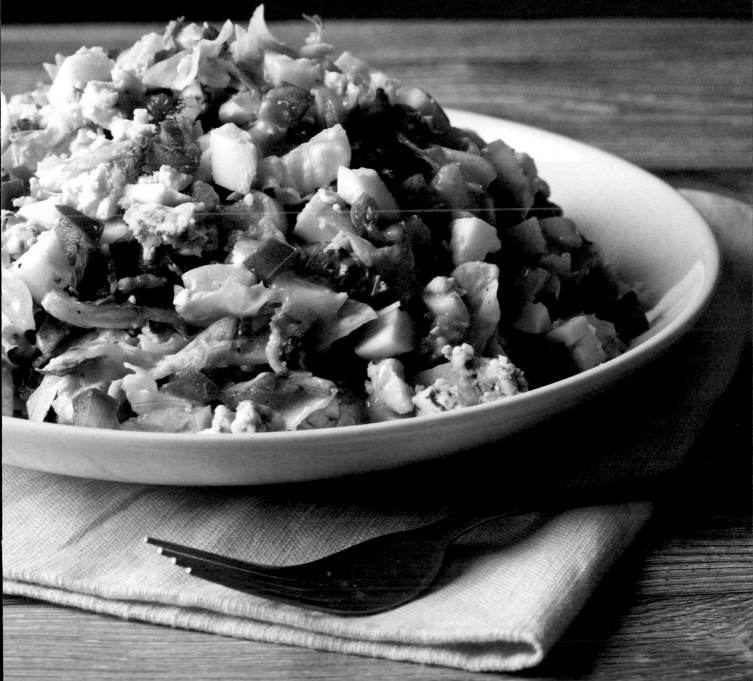

Lentil Soup

Makes 6 to 8 servings

2 tablespoons olive oil, divided

2 medium onions, chopped

1½ teaspoons salt

4 cloves garlic, minced

¼ cup tomato paste

1 teaspoon dried oregano

½ teaspoon dried basil

¼ teaspoon dried thyme

¼ teaspoon black pepper

½ cup dry sherry or white wine

8 cups vegetable broth

2 cups water

3 carrots, cut into ½-inch pieces

2 cups dried lentils, rinsed and sorted

½ cup chopped fresh parsley

1 tablespoon balsamic vinegar

1. Heat 1 tablespoon oil in large saucepan or Dutch oven over medium heat. Add onions; cook 10 minutes, stirring occasionally. Add remaining 1 tablespoon oil and salt; cook 10 minutes or until onions are golden brown, stirring frequently.

2. Add garlic; cook and stir 1 minute. Add tomato paste, oregano, basil, thyme and pepper; cook and stir 1 minute. Stir in sherry; cook 30 seconds, scraping up browned bits from bottom of saucepan.

3. Stir in broth, water, carrots and lentils; cover and bring to a boil over high heat. Reduce heat to medium-low; cook, partially covered, 30 minutes or until lentils are tender.

4. Remove from heat; stir in parsley and vinegar.

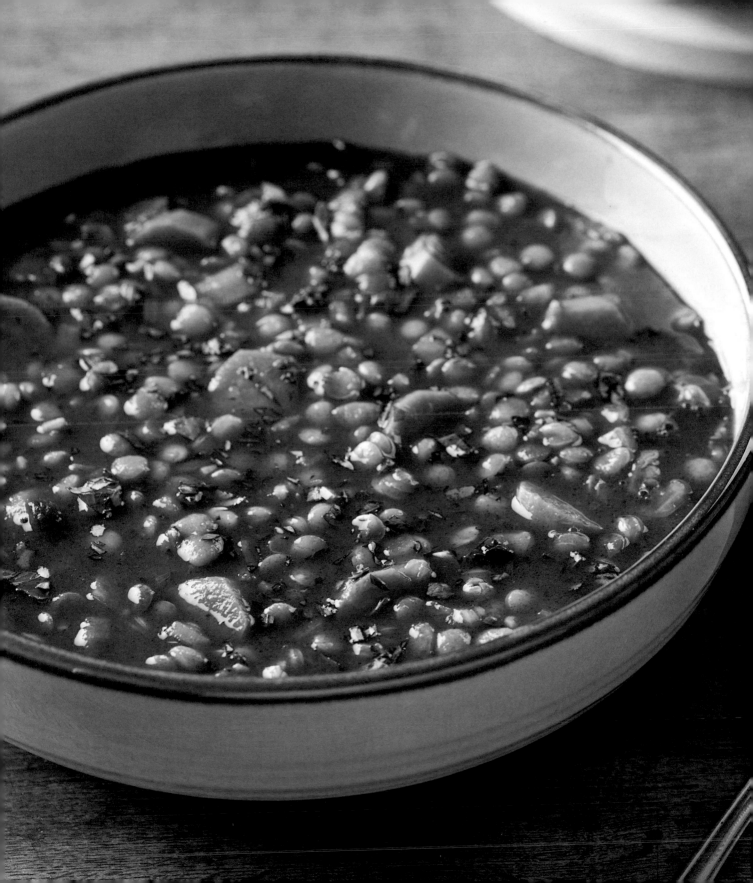

Broccoli & Cauliflower Salad

Makes 8 servings

1 package (about 12 ounces) bacon, chopped

2 cups mayonnaise

¼ cup sugar

¼ cup white or cider vinegar

4 cups chopped raw broccoli

4 cups coarsely chopped raw cauliflower

1½ cups (6 ounces) shredded Cheddar cheese

1 cup chopped red onion

1 cup dried cranberries or raisins (optional)

½ cup sunflower seeds (optional)

Salt and black pepper

1. Heat large skillet over medium heat. Add bacon; cook and stir until crisp. Remove from skillet with slotted spoon; drain on paper towel-lined plate.

2. Whisk mayonnaise, sugar and vinegar in large bowl. Stir in broccoli, cauliflower, cheese, onion and cranberries, if desired; mix well. Fold in bacon and sunflower seeds, if desired. Season with salt and pepper.

3. Serve immediately or cover and refrigerate until ready to serve.

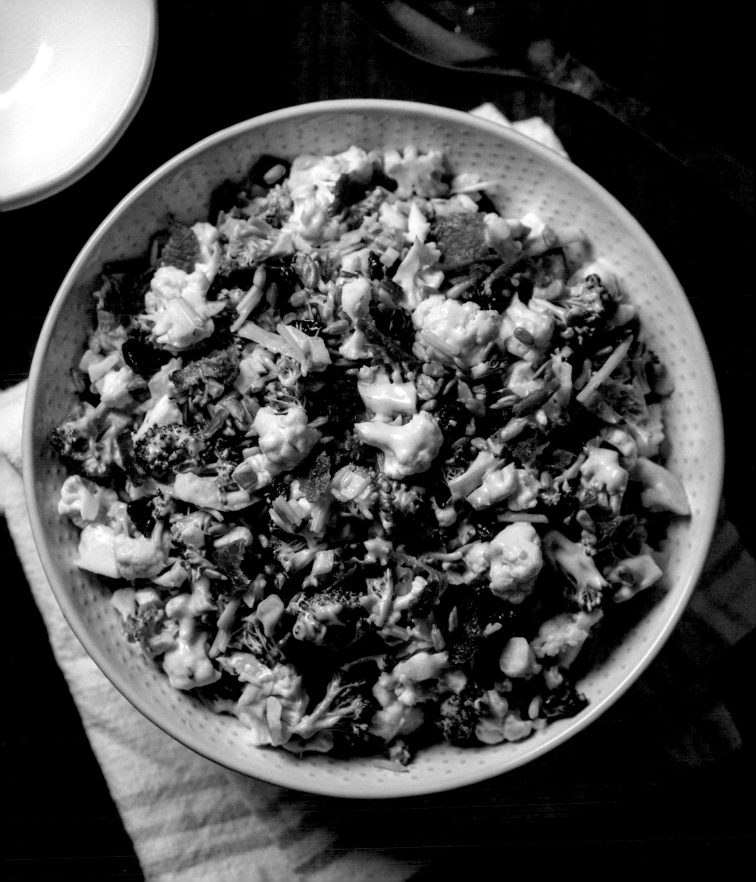

Edamame Peanut Slaw

Makes 8 cups (6 to 8 servings)

4 cups thinly sliced green
   cabbage

3 cups thinly sliced red cabbage
   (about ½ of a small head)

1 red bell pepper, thinly sliced

1 cup thawed frozen shelled
   edamame

3 green onions, thinly sliced

1 carrot, shredded or julienned

   Juice of 1 lime

2 tablespoons unseasoned rice
   vinegar

1 tablespoon toasted sesame oil

2 teaspoons salt

1 teaspoon sugar

1 teaspoon minced fresh ginger

1 cup roasted peanuts

1. Combine green cabbage, red cabbage, bell pepper, edamame, green onions and carrot in large bowl. Whisk lime juice, vinegar, oil, salt, sugar and ginger in small bowl until salt and sugar are dissolved.

2. Pour dressing over salad; mix well. Refrigerate until ready to serve. Stir in peanuts just before serving.

Note: This salad can be made at least one day ahead of time, but will even be good for several days. Store in a covered bowl or container and adjust the salt, lime juice and vinegar before serving. For crunchy peanuts, stir them in just before serving. They will also be fine if you stir them in early and let them sit. Their texture will be more crisp-tender than crisp, similar to the edamame.

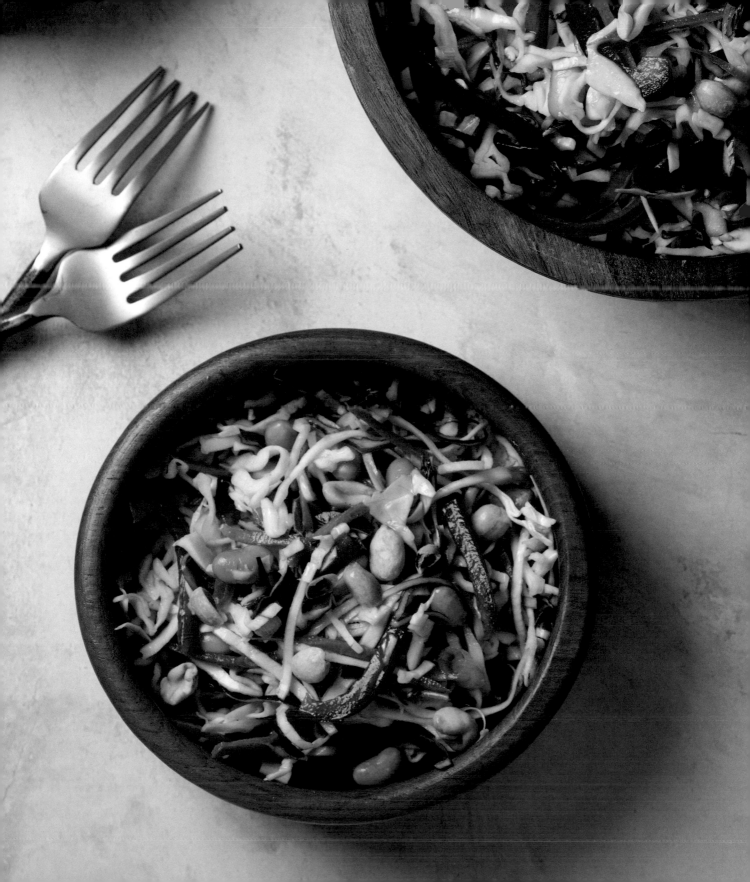

Coconut Cauliflower Cream Soup

Makes 6 servings

1 tablespoon coconut or
vegetable oil

1 medium onion, chopped

1 tablespoon minced garlic

1 tablespoon minced fresh
ginger

1 teaspoon salt

1 head cauliflower (1½ pounds),
cut into florets

2 cans (about 13 ounces each)
coconut milk, divided

1 cup water

1 teaspoon garam masala

½ teaspoon ground turmeric

Optional toppings: hot chili
oil, red pepper flakes and/or
chopped fresh cilantro

1. Heat oil in large saucepan over medium-high heat. Add onion; cook and stir 5 minutes or until softened. Add garlic, ginger and salt; cook and stir 30 seconds.

2. Add cauliflower, 1 can of coconut milk, water, garam masala and turmeric. Reduce heat to medium; cover and simmer 20 minutes or until cauliflower is very tender.

3. Remove from heat. Blend soup with immersion blender until smooth.* Return saucepan to medium heat; add 1 cup coconut milk. Cook and stir until heated through. Add additional coconut milk, if desired, to reach desired consistency. Serve with desired toppings.

Or blend soup in batches in blender or food processor.

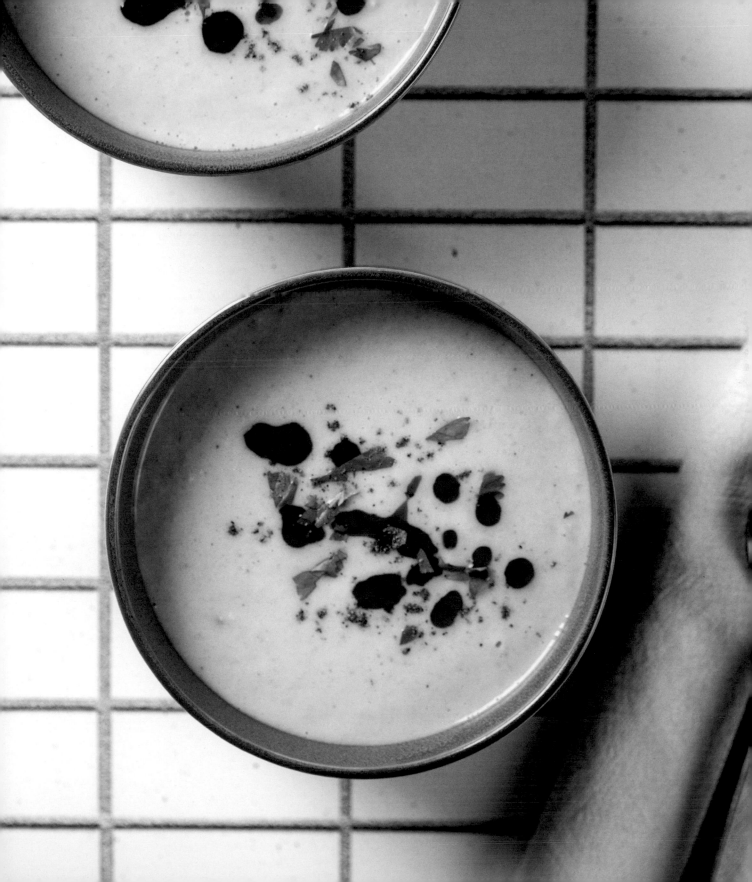

Green Goddess Cobb Salad

Makes 4 servings

Pickled Onions (recipe follows)

Dressing

1 cup mayonnaise

1 cup fresh Italian parsley leaves

1 cup baby arugula

¼ cup olive oil

3 tablespoons lemon juice

3 tablespoons minced fresh chives

2 tablespoons fresh tarragon leaves

1 clove garlic, minced

1 teaspoon Dijon mustard

½ teaspoon salt

⅛ teaspoon black pepper

Salad

4 cups Italian salad blend (romaine and radicchio)

2 cups chopped stemmed kale

2 cups baby arugula

2 avocados, halved and sliced

2 tomatoes, cut into wedges

2 cups grilled or roasted chicken breast strips or cut-up rotisserie chicken

1 cup chopped crisp-cooked bacon

4 hard-cooked eggs (see Tip on page 50), cut in half

1. Prepare Pickled Onions.

2. For dressing, combine mayonnaise, parsley, 1 cup arugula, oil, lemon juice, chives, tarragon, garlic, mustard, ½ teaspoon salt and pepper in blender or food processor; blend until smooth, stopping to scrape side once or twice. Transfer to jar; refrigerate until ready to use. Just before serving, thin dressing with 1 to 2 tablespoons water, if necessary, to reach desired consistency.

3. For salad, combine salad blend, kale, 2 cups arugula and pickled onions in large bowl; divide among four serving bowls. Top each salad with avocados, tomatoes, chicken, bacon and 2 egg halves. Drizzle each with ¼ cup dressing.

Pickled Onions: Combine 1 cup thinly sliced red onion, ½ cup white wine vinegar, ¼ cup water, 2 teaspoons sugar and 1 teaspoon salt in large glass jar. Seal jar; shake well. Refrigerate at least 1 hour or up to 1 week.

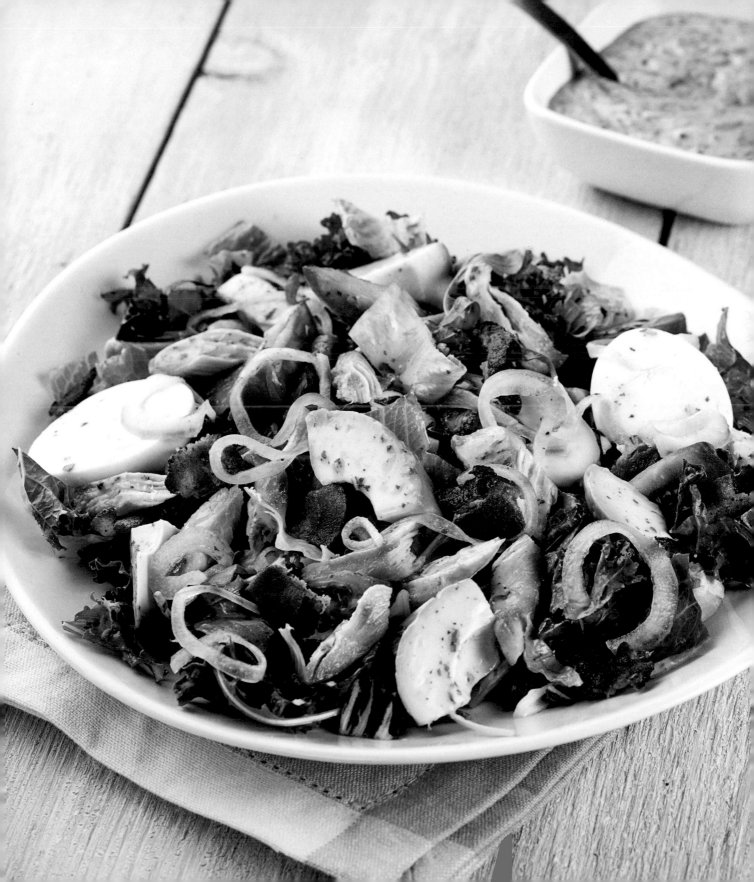

Baked Potato Soup

Makes 6 to 8 servings (8 cups)

3 medium russet potatoes (about 1 pound)

¼ cup (½ stick) butter

1 large onion, chopped

4 cups chicken or vegetable broth

1¾ cups instant mashed potato flakes

1 cup water

1 cup half-and-half

1 teaspoon salt

½ teaspoon dried basil

½ teaspoon dried thyme

¼ teaspoon black pepper

1 cup (4 ounces) shredded Cheddar cheese

4 slices bacon, crisp-cooked and chopped

1 green onion, chopped

1. Preheat oven to 400°F. Scrub potatoes and prick in several places with fork. Place in baking pan; bake 1 hour. Cool completely; peel and cut into ½-inch cubes. (Potatoes can be prepared several days in advance; refrigerate until ready to use.)

2. Melt butter in large saucepan or Dutch oven over medium heat. Add onion; cook and stir 5 minutes or until softened. Stir in broth, mashed potato flakes, water, half-and-half, salt, basil, thyme and pepper; bring to a boil over medium-high heat. Reduce heat to medium; cook 5 minutes.

3. Stir in baked potato cubes; cook 10 to 15 minutes or until soup is thickened and heated through. Ladle into bowls; top with cheese, bacon and green onion.

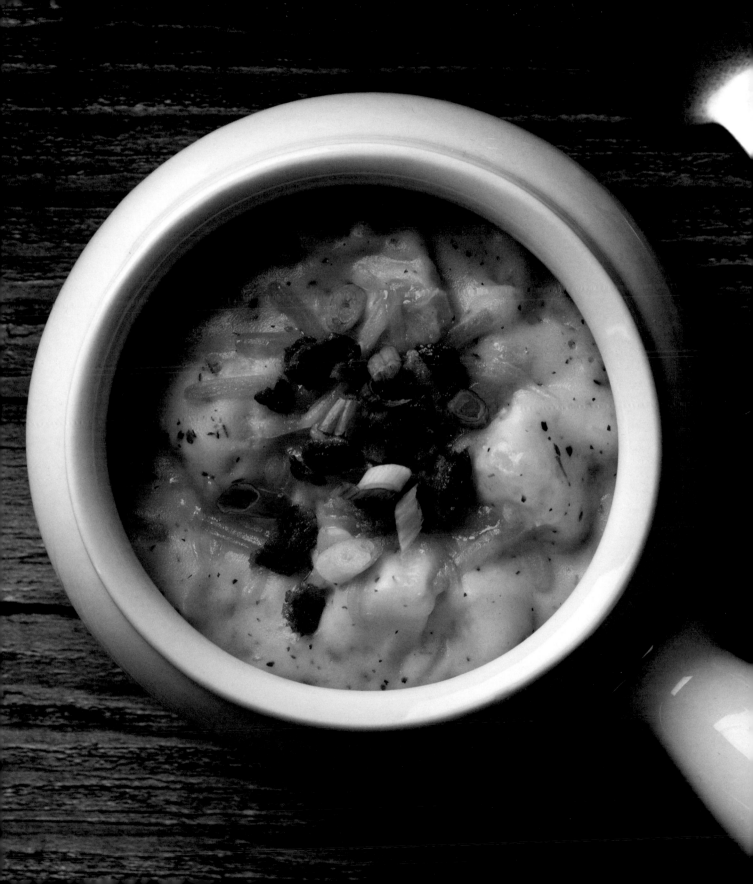

Chicken Satay Salad

Makes 4 servings

¼ cup plus 2 tablespoons Thai peanut sauce, divided

2 tablespoons lime juice

1 tablespoon unseasoned rice vinegar

3 teaspoons toasted sesame oil, divided

1 pound chicken tenders, cut in half lengthwise

4 cups chopped romaine lettuce

1 red bell pepper, thinly sliced

1 cup shredded carrots

1 cup sliced Persian* or seedless cucumbers

¼ cup chopped fresh cilantro

¼ cup peanuts, chopped

Persian cucumbers are similar to English cucumbers; they have fewer seeds and contain less water than traditional cucumbers, which gives them a sweeter flavor and crunchier texture. These smaller cucumbers can be found in packages in the produce section of the supermarket.

1. Whisk ¼ cup peanut sauce, lime juice, vinegar and 1 teaspoon oil in large bowl until smooth and well blended. Set aside.

2. Heat remaining 2 teaspoons oil in large nonstick skillet over medium-high heat. Add chicken; cook and stir 4 minutes or until chicken is no longer pink. Remove from heat. Add remaining 2 tablespoons peanut sauce; stir to coat chicken.

3. Add lettuce, bell pepper, carrots and cucumbers to dressing in large bowl; toss to coat.

4. Divide salad evenly among four plates. Top with chicken, cilantro and peanuts.

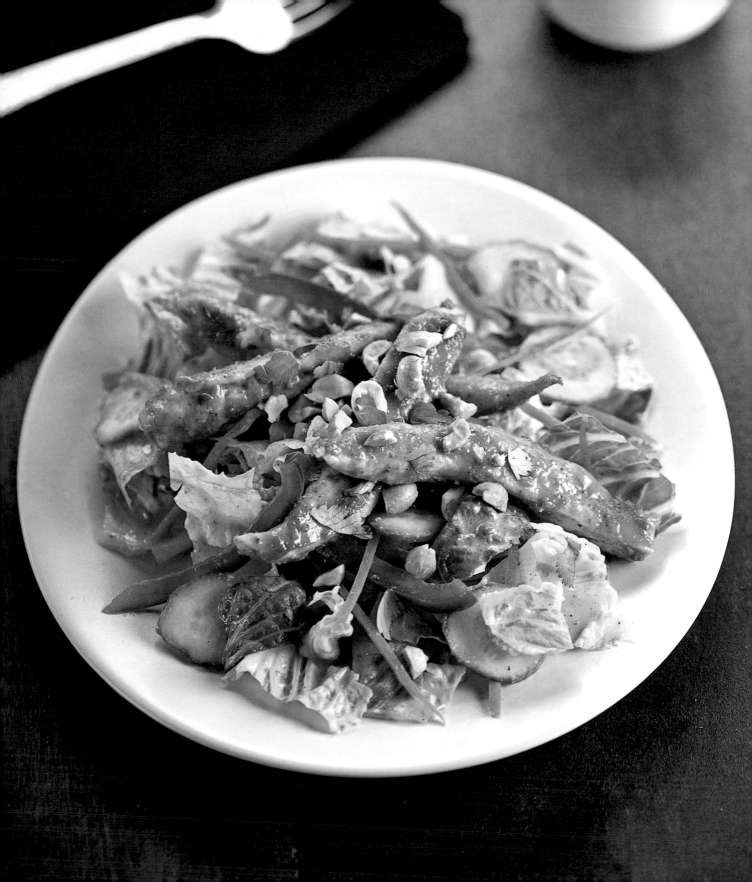

Middle Eastern Chicken Soup

Makes 4 servings

1 can (about 14 ounces) chicken broth

2½ cups water

1 can (about 15 ounces) chickpeas, rinsed and drained

1 cup chopped cooked chicken

1 small onion, chopped

1 carrot, chopped

1 clove garlic, minced

1 teaspoon salt

1 teaspoon dried oregano

1 teaspoon ground cumin

1 package (5 ounces) baby spinach

⅛ teaspoon black pepper

1. Combine broth, water, chickpeas, chicken, onion, carrot, garlic, salt, oregano and cumin in medium saucepan. Bring to a boil over high heat. Reduce heat to medium-low; cover and simmer 15 minutes.

2. Stir in spinach and pepper; simmer, uncovered, 2 minutes or until spinach is wilted.

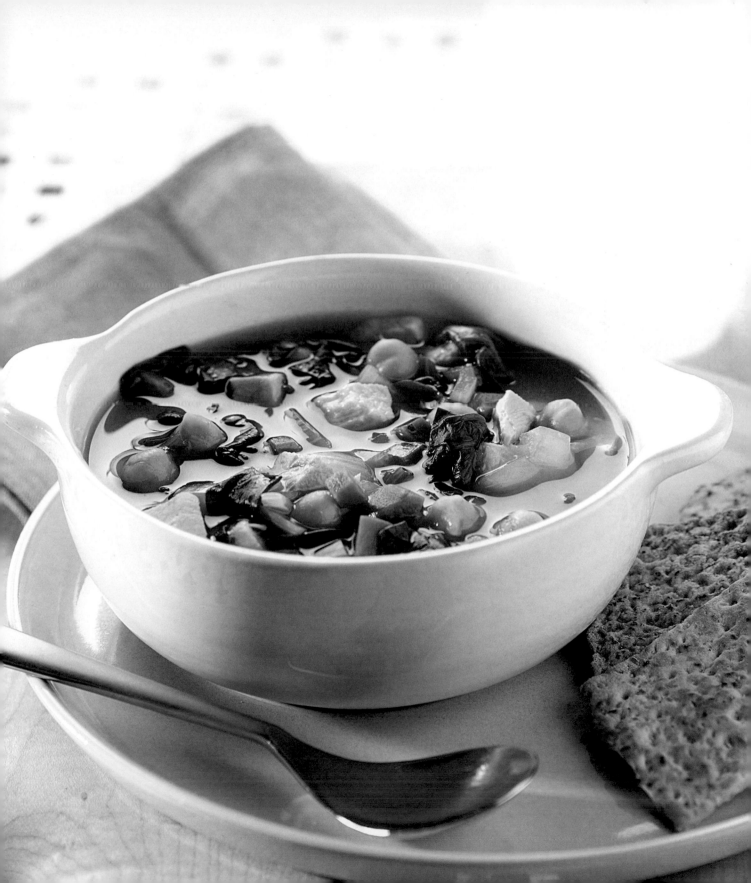

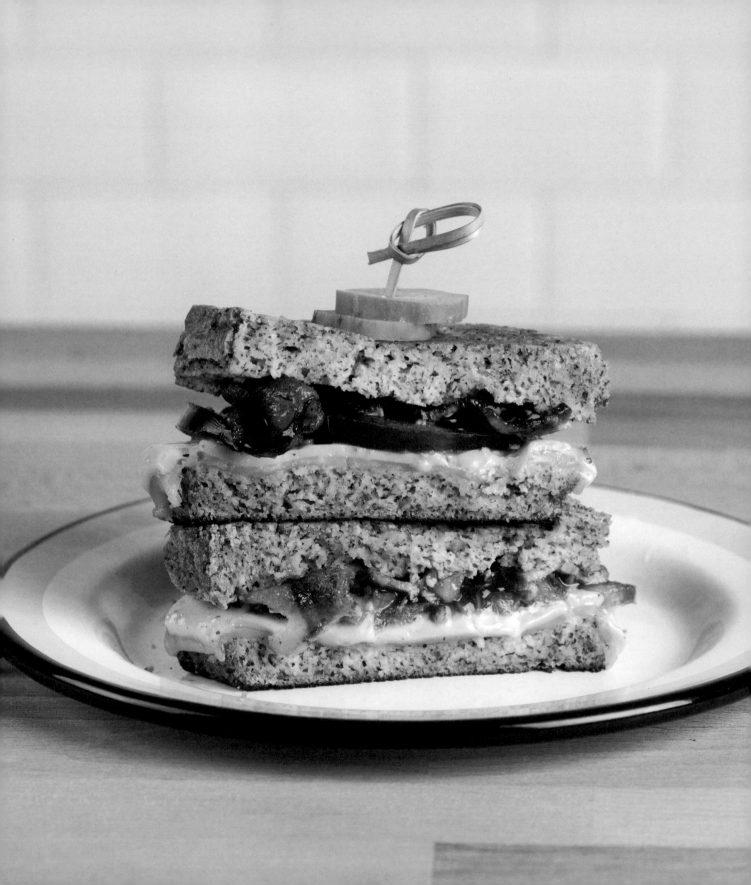

pizzas, wraps *and* sandwiches

Bacon-Tomato Grilled Cheese

Makes 4 servings

8 slices bacon, cut in half

4 slices sharp Cheddar cheese

4 slices Gouda cheese

4 tomato slices

8 slices Almond Flour Quick Bread (page 168) or purchased gluten-free bread

1 tablespoon butter

1. Cook bacon in large skillet over medium heat until crisp. Remove from skillet; drain on paper towel-lined plate. Drain fat from skillet; wipe out skillet with paper towels.

2. Layer 1 slice of Cheddar cheese, 1 slice of Gouda cheese, 1 tomato slice and 2 bacon slices between 2 bread slices.

3. Melt 1 tablespoon butter in same skillet over medium heat. Add sandwiches; cook 3 to 4 minutes or until bottoms are toasted. Flip sandwiches. Reduce heat to medium-low; cover and cook 3 to 4 minutes or until bottoms are toasted and cheese is melted.

Spinach & Mushroom Cauliflower Pizza

Makes 6 to 8 servings

2 teaspoons vegetable oil

1 head cauliflower (1½ pounds)

¾ cup almond flour

½ cup shredded Parmesan cheese

1½ cups (6 ounces) shredded mozzarella cheese, divided

1 teaspoon salt

1 clove garlic, minced

½ teaspoon dried oregano

Black pepper

1 egg

1 cup pizza sauce or marinara sauce

1 tablespoon chopped garlic

1 tomato, thinly sliced

1 cup sliced mushrooms

½ cup baby spinach

1. Preheat oven to 425°F. Grease large sheet pan with oil.

2. Break cauliflower into florets. Working in batches, pulse cauliflower in food processor until finely chopped. Measure 4 cups; place in large bowl. Reserve remaining cauliflower for another use. Add almond flour, Parmesan cheese, ½ cup mozzarella cheese, salt, 1 clove garlic and oregano. Season with pepper; mix well. Add egg; mix with hands until thoroughly blended.

3. Turn out onto prepared sheet pan; pat into 11-inch circle, building up a slight rim around edge. Bake 20 minutes. (Crust will be firm and browned around edges.)

4. Remove crust from oven. *Increase oven temperature to 450°F.* Spread sauce over crust to within ½ inch of edges. Top with garlic; spread evenly. Sprinkle with ½ cup mozzarella cheese; top evenly with tomato slices, mushrooms and spinach; sprinkle with remaining ½ cup mozzarella cheese.

5. Bake 7 to 10 minutes or until cheese is bubbly and browned in spots. Cut into wedges to serve.

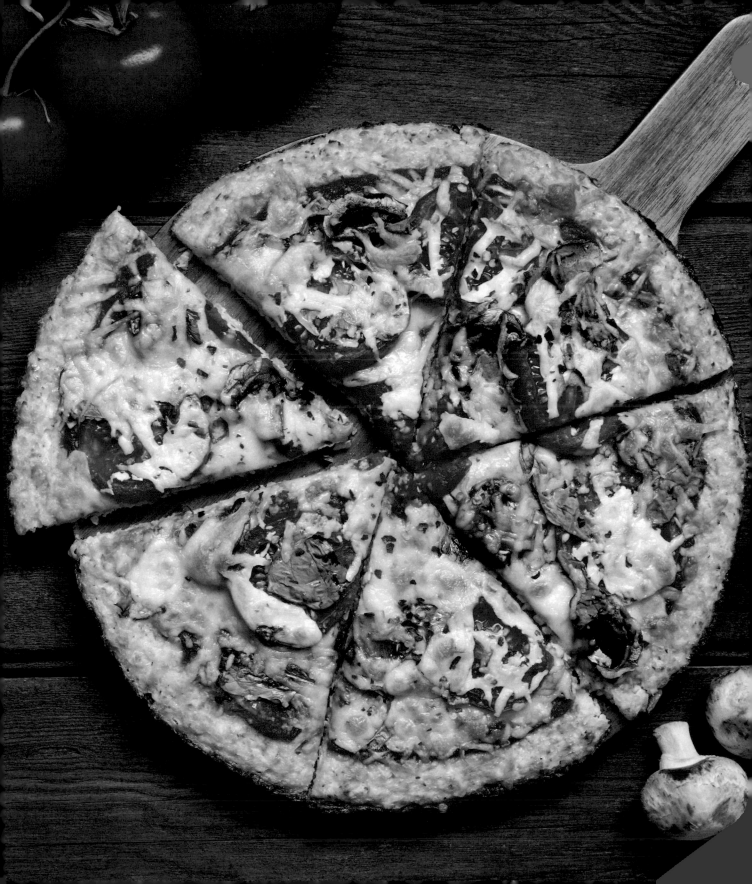

Niçoise Salad Wraps

Makes 2 servings

8 cups water

2 tablespoons salt

½ cup bite-size green bean pieces

2 new red potatoes, each cut into 8 wedges

2 tablespoons vinaigrette, divided

1 egg

2 cups watercress leaves

4 ounces water-packed albacore tuna, drained and flaked (about ½ cup)

8 niçoise olives, pitted and halved

3 cherry tomatoes, quartered

2 (10-inch) gluten-free tortillas

1. Bring water and salt to a boil in large saucepan over high heat. Add green beans and potatoes. Reduce heat to low; simmer 6 minutes or until tender. Remove vegetables with slotted spoon; plunge in ice water to stop cooking. Drain on paper towels. Transfer to medium bowl; toss with 1 tablespoon vinaigrette.

2. Return water to a boil. Add egg; reduce heat to medium and simmer 12 minutes. Drain and run under cold water until cool. Peel and cut into 8 wedges.

3. Add watercress, tuna, olives, tomatoes and remaining 1 tablespoon vinaigrette to vegetables; toss gently.

4. Heat tortillas in nonstick skillet over medium-high heat, turning when softened. Place on plates. Divide salad between tortillas; top with egg wedges. Roll up tortillas to enclose filling.

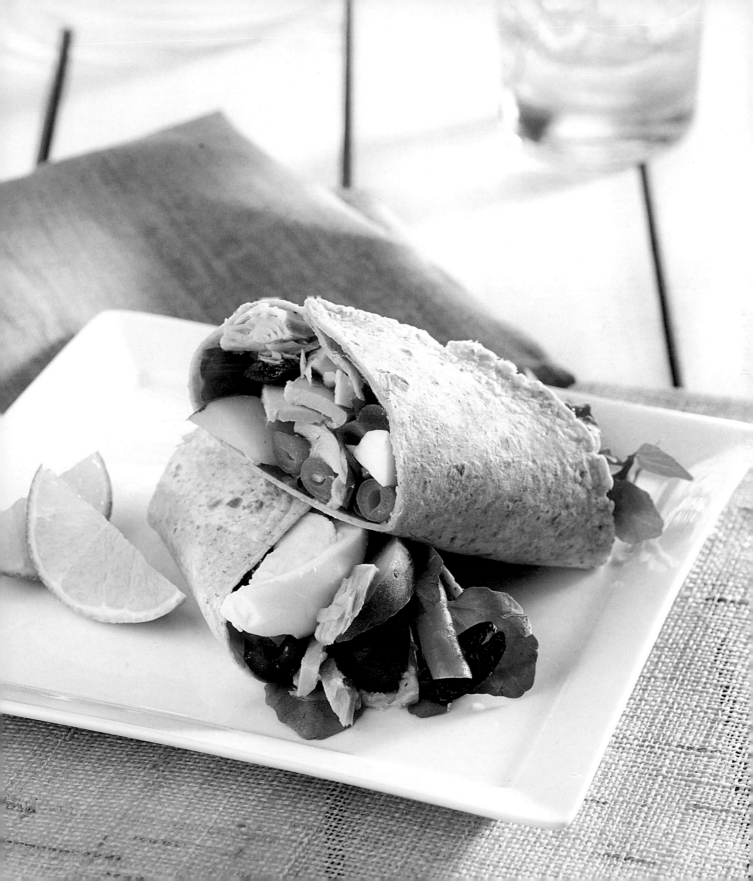

Quinoa Crust Cheese Pizza

Makes 4 servings

1 cup uncooked quinoa

⅓ cup water, plus additional for soaking

1 teaspoon baking powder

¾ teaspoon kosher salt

1 tablespoon olive oil, plus additional for serving

½ cup marinara sauce

1 ball (8 ounces) fresh mozzarella cheese, cut into ¼-inch-thick slices

Slivered fresh basil, flaky sea salt and black pepper (optional)

1. Place quinoa in medium bowl; cover with 1 inch of water. Cover and let soak 8 hours or overnight. Drain and rinse well in fine-mesh strainer.

2. Combine soaked quinoa, ⅓ cup water, baking powder and salt in bowl of food processor. Process 2 minutes or until completely smooth, stopping occasionally to scrape down sides of bowl as needed.

3. Preheat oven to 450°F. Line bottom of 10-inch springform pan with foil. Brush with 1 tablespoon oil. Attach sides of pan. Pour quinoa mixture in pan, spreading evenly with spatula. Bake 10 to 12 minutes or until crust is golden on sides and bottom.

4. Remove pan from oven; place on baking sheet. Remove sides of pan. Spread marinara sauce evenly over crust; top with cheese. Bake 10 minutes or until cheese is melted.

5. Slide pizza onto large cutting board. Top with basil and drizzle with additional oil. Sprinkle with sea salt and pepper, if desired. Slice and serve immediately.

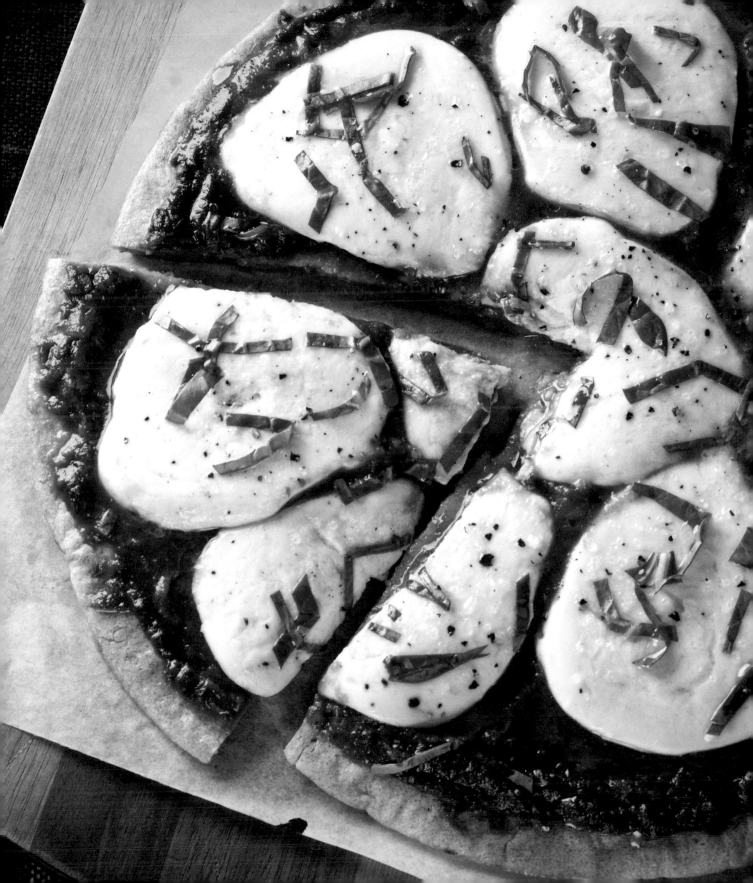

Tortilla Pizza Wedges

Makes 4 servings

4 (6-inch) corn tortillas

2 teaspoons vegetable oil

1 cup frozen corn, thawed

1 cup thinly sliced mushrooms

½ cup chopped onion

¼ cup pasta sauce, pizza sauce or thick and chunky salsa

1 to 2 teaspoons chopped jalapeño pepper

½ teaspoon dried oregano

½ cup (2 ounces) shredded pepper-jack or mozzarella cheese

1. Preheat oven to 450°F. Place tortillas on baking sheet. Bake 4 minutes or until edges begin to brown.

2. Heat oil in medium skillet over medium heat. Add corn, mushrooms and onion; cook and stir 4 to 5 minutes or until tender.

3. Combine pasta sauce, jalapeño and oregano in small bowl. Spread evenly over tortillas. Top evenly with vegetables. Sprinkle with cheese.

4. Bake 4 to 5 minutes or until cheese is melted and pizzas are heated through. Cut each pizza into four wedges.

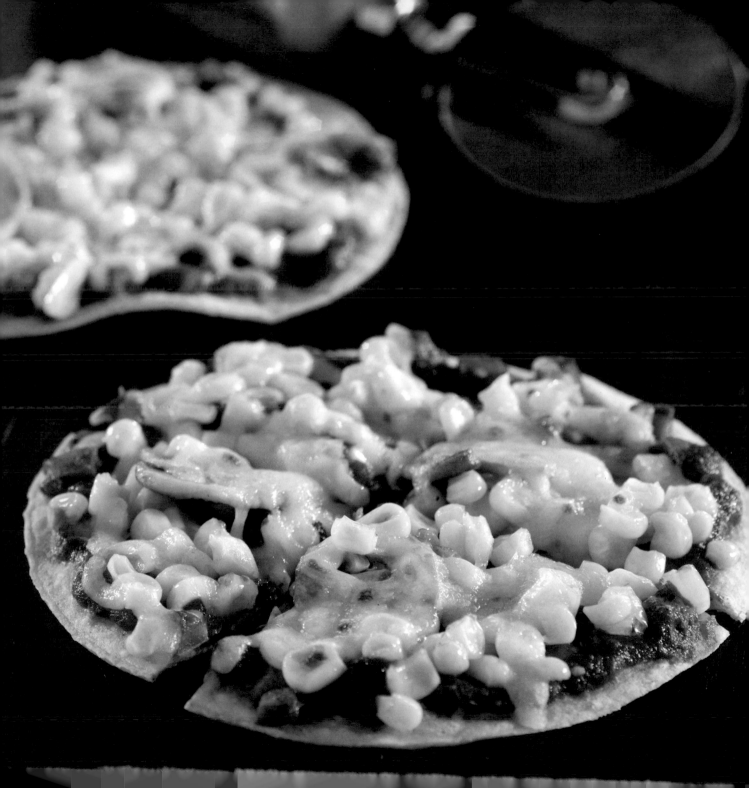

Spinach Veggie Wraps

Makes 4 servings

Pico de Gallo

- 1 cup finely chopped tomatoes (about 2 small)
- ½ teaspoon salt
- ¼ cup chopped white onion
- 2 tablespoons minced jalapeño pepper
- 2 tablespoons chopped fresh cilantro
- 1 teaspoon lime juice

Guacamole

- 2 large ripe avocados
- ¼ cup finely chopped red onion
- 2 tablespoons chopped fresh cilantro
- 2 teaspoons fresh lime juice
- ½ teaspoon salt

Wraps

- 4 (10-inch) gluten-free tortillas
- 2 cups baby spinach
- 1 cup sliced mushrooms
- 1 cup shredded Asiago cheese
  Salsa

1. For pico de gallo, combine tomatoes and ½ teaspoon salt in fine-mesh strainer; set over bowl to drain 15 minutes. Combine drained tomatoes, white onion, jalapeño, 2 tablespoons cilantro and 1 teaspoon lime juice in medium bowl; mix well.

2. For guacamole, combine avocados, red onion, 2 tablespoons cilantro, 2 teaspoons lime juice and ½ teaspoon salt in medium bowl; mash with fork to desired consistency.

3. For wraps, spread ¼ cup guacamole on each tortilla. Layer each with ½ cup spinach, ¼ cup mushrooms, ¼ cup cheese and ¼ cup pico de gallo. Roll up; serve with salsa.

Tip: To make these wraps super easy, purchase premade pico de gallo and guacamole from the grocery store.

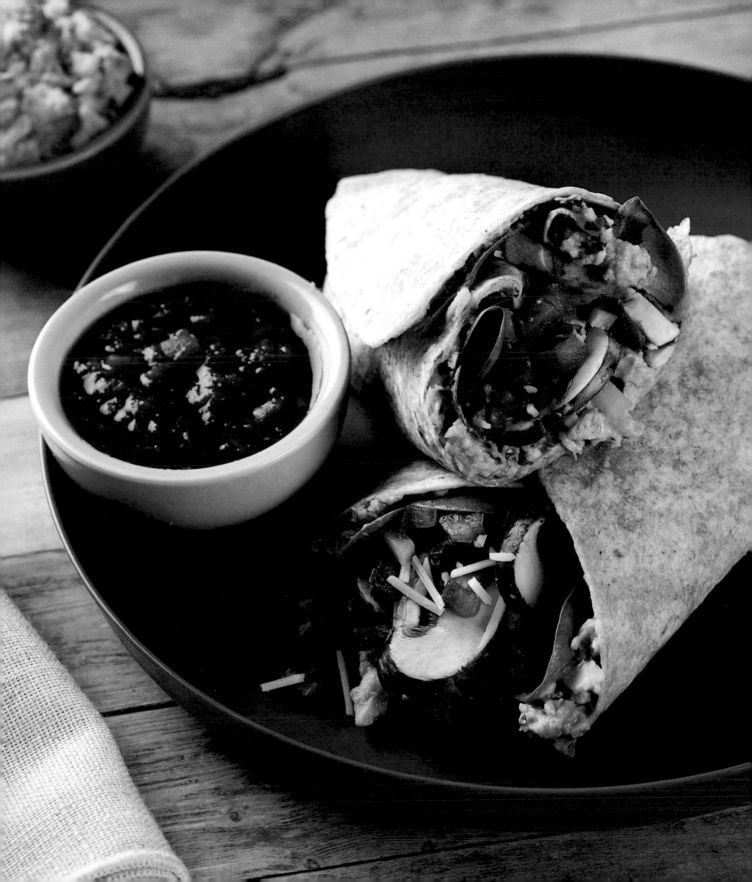

Chicken Pesto Pizzas

Makes 6 servings

1 package (10.6 ounces) prepared gluten-free pizza crusts (2 crusts)

⅓ cup pesto sauce

1 cup shredded or chopped cooked chicken

1 plum tomato, thinly sliced

½ cup baby spinach, coarsely chopped

1 cup (4 ounces) shredded mozzarella cheese

1. Preheat oven to 375°F.

2. Place crusts on pizza pans or baking sheets. Spread pesto evenly over crusts; layer with chicken, tomato slices, spinach and cheese.

3. Bake 12 to 14 minutes or until cheese is melted and crusts are golden brown.

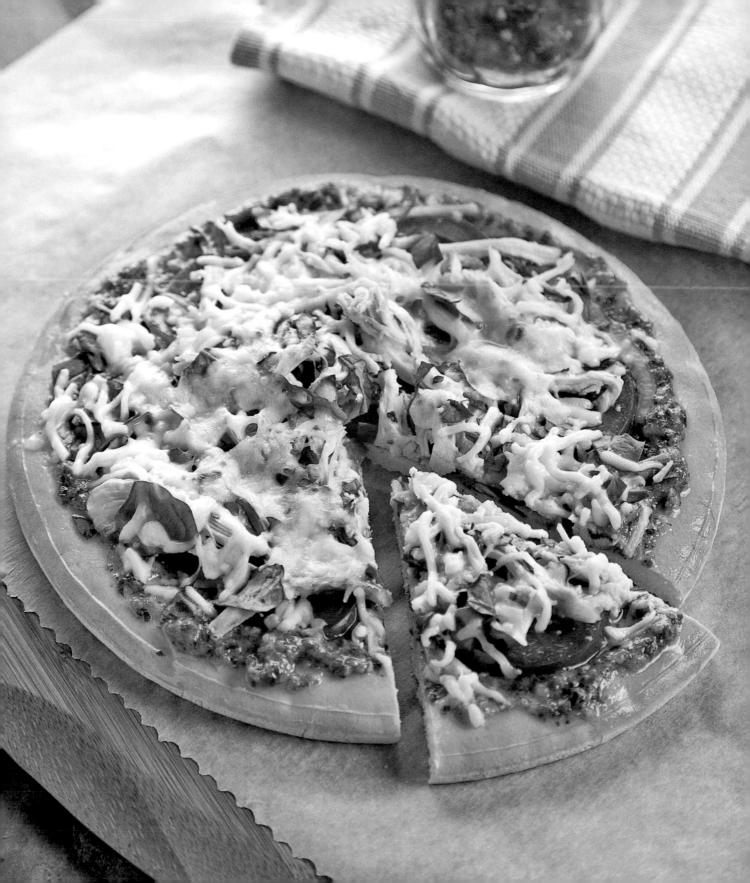

Tuna Melt

Makes 4 servings

- ¾ cup mayonnaise
- 2 teaspoons lemon juice
- 1 teaspoon salt
- ⅛ teaspoon black pepper
- 1 can (12 ounces) solid white albacore tuna, drained
- 1 can (12 ounces) chunk light tuna, drained
- 1 stalk celery, finely chopped (about ½ cup)
- ¼ cup minced red onion
- 8 slices Almond Flour Quick Bread (page 168) or purchased gluten-free bread
- 8 slices Cheddar or American cheese
- 2 tablespoons butter

  Optional toppings: tomato slices, red onion rings, pickles and/or sliced avocados

1. Combine mayonnaise, lemon juice, salt and pepper in large bowl. Add tuna, celery and onion; mix well.

2. Divide tuna mixture among bread slices; top each with cheese. Heat 1 tablespoon butter in large skillet over medium heat until melted. Add half of sandwiches; cover and cook until bread is toasted and cheese is melted. Repeat with remaining butter and sandwiches. Serve with desired toppings.

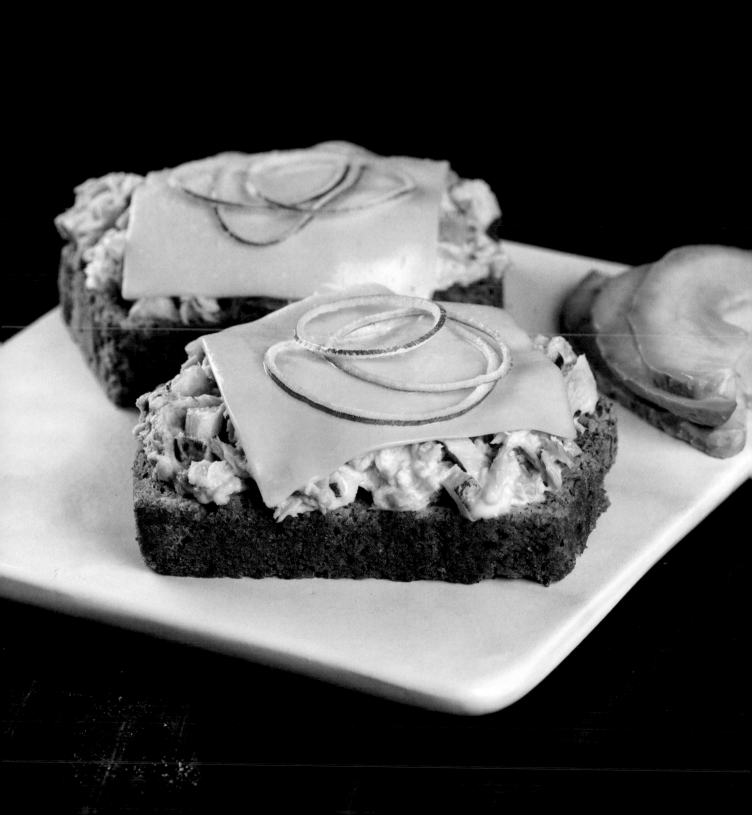

Thai-Inspired Cauliflower Pizza

Makes 8 servings

Crust

2 teaspoons vegetable oil

1 head cauliflower (1½ pounds)

¾ cup almond flour

½ cup shredded Parmesan cheese

½ cup (2 ounces) shredded
    mozzarella cheese

1 teaspoon salt

1 egg

Toppings

½ cup Thai peanut sauce

½ cup thinly sliced red onion

1 carrot, chopped

1 cup (4 ounces) shredded
    mozzarella

1 cup coleslaw mix*

¼ cup chopped fresh cilantro

1 tablespoon lime juice

⅛ teaspoon salt

3 tablespoons chopped roasted
    unsalted peanuts

**Or substitute ¾ cup shredded
green or napa cabbage and ¼ cup
shredded carrot.*

1. Preheat oven to 425°F. Grease large sheet pan with oil or line with parchment paper.

2. Break cauliflower into florets. Working in batches, pulse cauliflower in food processor until finely chopped. Measure 4 cups; reserve remaining cauliflower for another use. Place in large bowl. Add almond flour, Parmesan cheese, ½ cup mozzarella cheese and 1 teaspoon salt; mix well. Add egg; mix with hands until thoroughly blended.

3. Turn out onto prepared sheet pan; pat into 11-inch circle. Bake 20 minutes. (Crust will be firm and browned around edges.)

4. Remove crust from oven. Spread sauce over crust to within ½ inch of edge. Sprinkle with onion, carrot and 1 cup mozzarella cheese. Bake 7 to 10 minutes or until cheese is melted and browned in spots.

5. Meanwhile, combine coleslaw mix, cilantro, lime juice and ⅛ teaspoon salt in small bowl. Stir in peanuts. Spread over pizza; cut into wedges to serve.

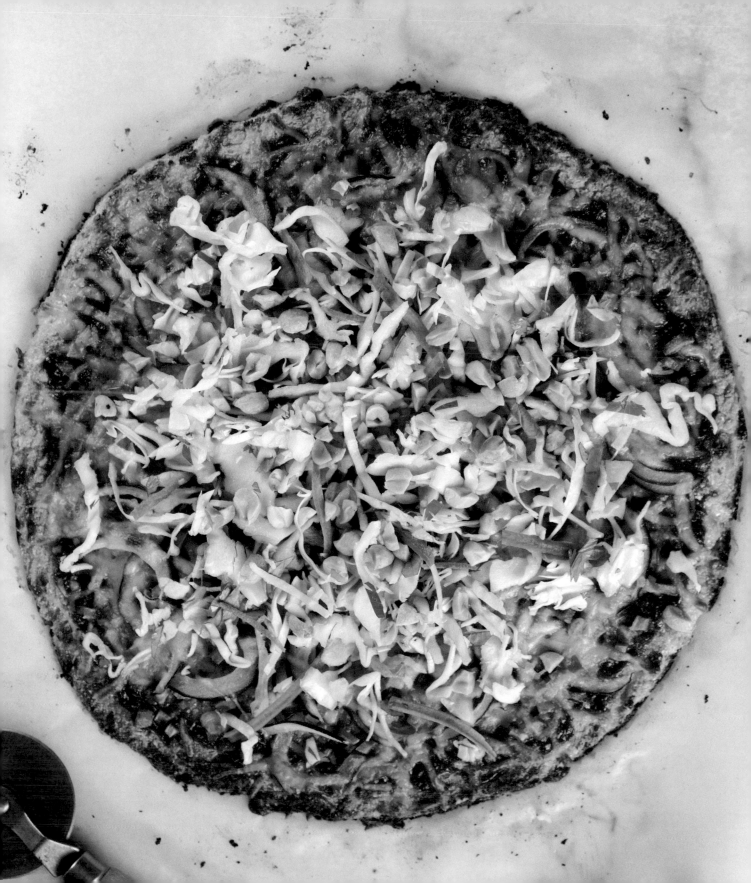

Black Bean & Bell Pepper Burritos

Makes 8 servings

2 teaspoons canola oil

2 cups diced red, yellow and/or green bell peppers

1 cup chopped onion

1 can (about 15 ounces) black beans, rinsed and drained

¾ cup salsa

2 teaspoons chili powder

½ teaspoon salt

½ teaspoon ground cumin

8 (8-inch) gluten-free tortillas, warmed

1 cup (4 ounces) shredded Cheddar or Mexican cheese blend

½ cup chopped fresh cilantro

1. Heat oil in large nonstick skillet over medium heat. Add bell peppers and onion; cook and stir 3 to 4 minutes. Stir in beans, salsa, chili powder, salt and cumin; cook and stir 5 to 8 minutes or until vegetables are tender and sauce is thickened.

2. Spoon about ⅔ cup bean mixture down center of each tortilla. Top with cheese and cilantro. Fold up about 1 inch of bottom and top of tortilla; roll up from one side to enclose filling.

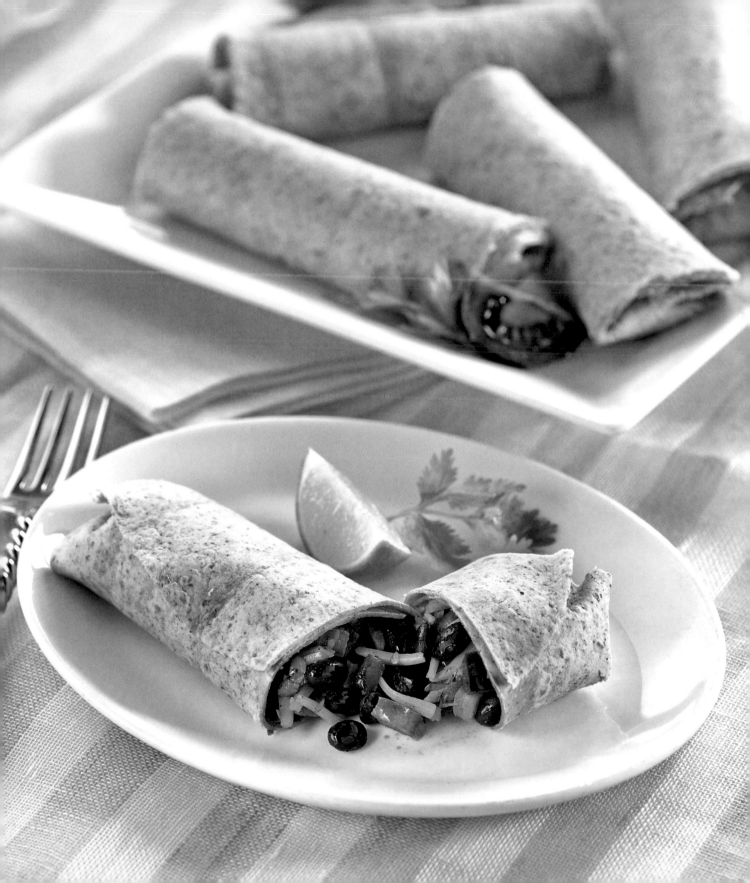

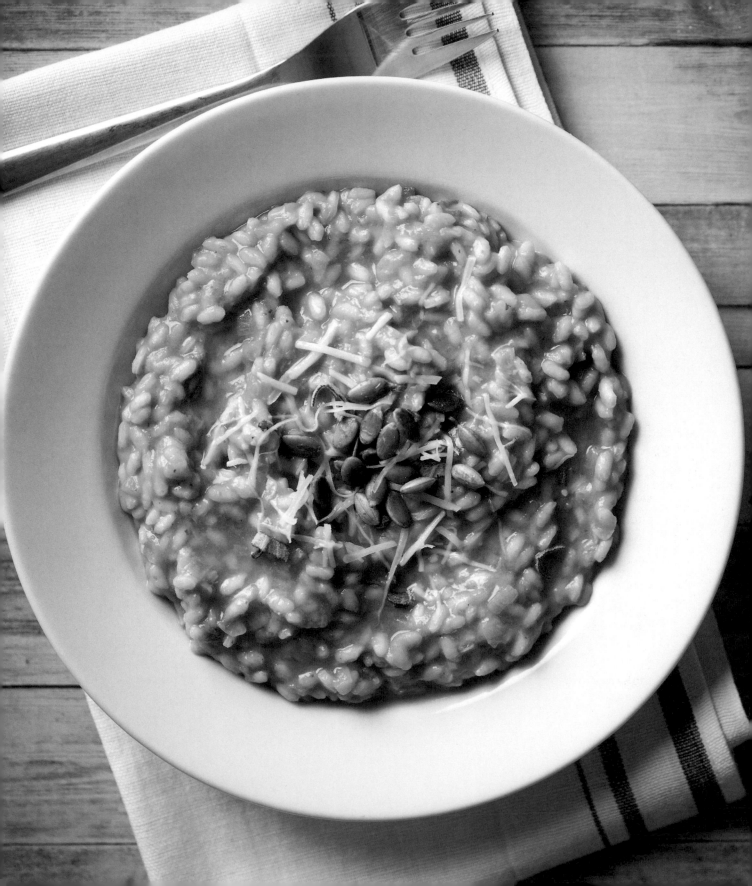

pasta *and* rice

Pumpkin Risotto
Makes 4 servings

4 cups vegetable broth

5 whole fresh sage leaves

¼ teaspoon ground nutmeg

2 tablespoons butter

1 tablespoon olive oil

1 onion, finely chopped

2 cloves garlic, minced

1½ cups uncooked arborio rice

½ cup dry white wine

1 teaspoon salt

Black pepper

1 can (15 ounces) pumpkin purée

½ cup shredded Parmesan cheese, plus additional for serving

2 tablespoons chopped fresh sage, divided

¼ cup roasted pumpkin seeds (pepitas) or chopped toasted walnuts or pecans

1. Combine broth, whole sage leaves and nutmeg in small saucepan; bring to a boil over high heat. Reduce heat to low to maintain a simmer.

2. Heat butter and oil in large saucepan over medium-high heat. Add onion; cook and stir 5 minutes or until softened. Add garlic; cook and stir 30 seconds. Add rice; cook 2 to 3 minutes or until rice appears translucent, stirring frequently to coat with butter. Add wine, salt and pepper; cook until most of liquid is absorbed.

3. Add broth mixture, ½ cup at a time, stirring frequently until broth is absorbed before adding next ½ cup (discard whole sage leaves). Stir in pumpkin when about 1 cup broth remains. Add remaining broth; cook until rice is al dente, stirring constantly. (If needed, add water by ½ cupfuls and continue to stir until rice is al dente.)

4. Remove from heat; stir in ½ cup cheese and 1 tablespoon chopped sage. Cover and let stand 5 minutes. Top each serving with 1 tablespoon pumpkin seeds, remaining chopped sage and additional cheese.

Classic Macaroni & Cheese

Makes 8 servings (about 8 cups)

1 package (12 ounces) uncooked gluten-free elbow macaroni

1 can (12 ounces) evaporated milk

2 tablespoons butter

1 teaspoon salt

⅛ teaspoon black pepper

4 cups (16 ounces) shredded Colby-Jack cheese

1. Cook pasta in large saucepan of salted boiling water 2 minutes less than package directions for al dente. Drain and return to saucepan, reserving 1 cup pasta water.

2. Add evaporated milk, butter, salt and pepper to pasta; cook over medium heat until butter melts. Add cheese by handfuls, stirring until well blended after each addition, adding pasta water ¼ cup at a time if needed until sauce is creamy and cheese is melted.

Tip: To turn this easy pasta into a hearty meal, stir in cooked frozen peas, steamed broccoli or carrots and canned tuna or chopped cooked chicken.

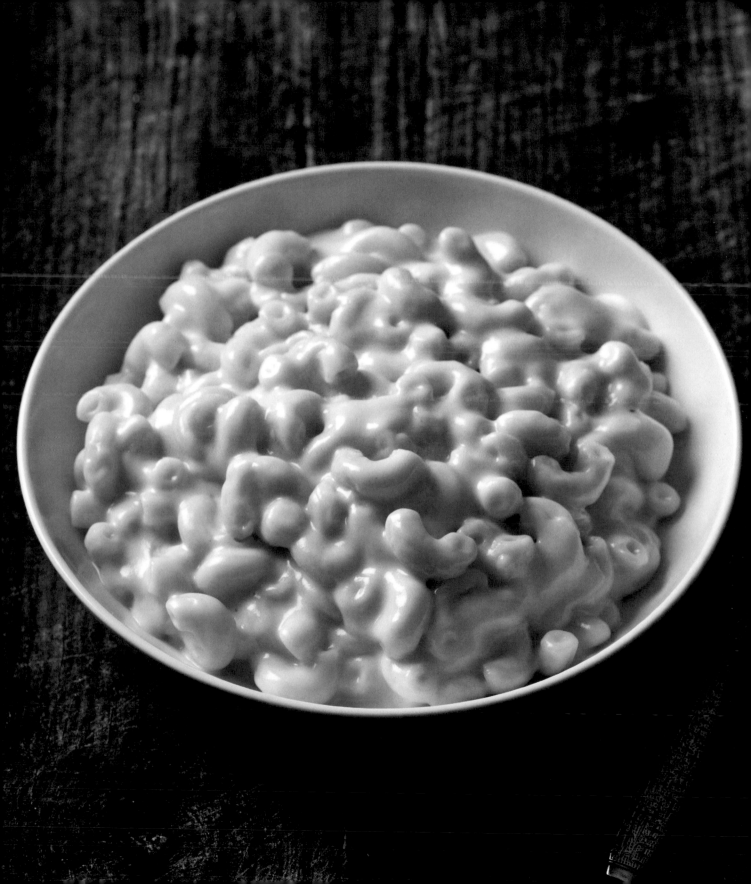

Brown Rice with Cranberries & Walnuts

Makes 4 to 6 servings

4 cups vegetable broth

1½ cups uncooked brown rice or brown basmati rice

1 teaspoon salt

½ cup dried cranberries

¼ teaspoon ground cinnamon

2 teaspoons olive oil

½ cup coarsely chopped walnuts

1. Combine broth, rice and salt in large saucepan. Bring to a boil over high heat. Reduce heat; cover and simmer 20 minutes.

2. Stir in cranberries and cinnamon; cover and simmer 20 to 25 minutes or until rice is tender.

3. Meanwhile, heat oil in medium skillet over medium heat. Add walnuts; cook and stir 3 to 4 minutes or until lightly browned. Drain on paper towel-lined plate. Sprinkle over rice.

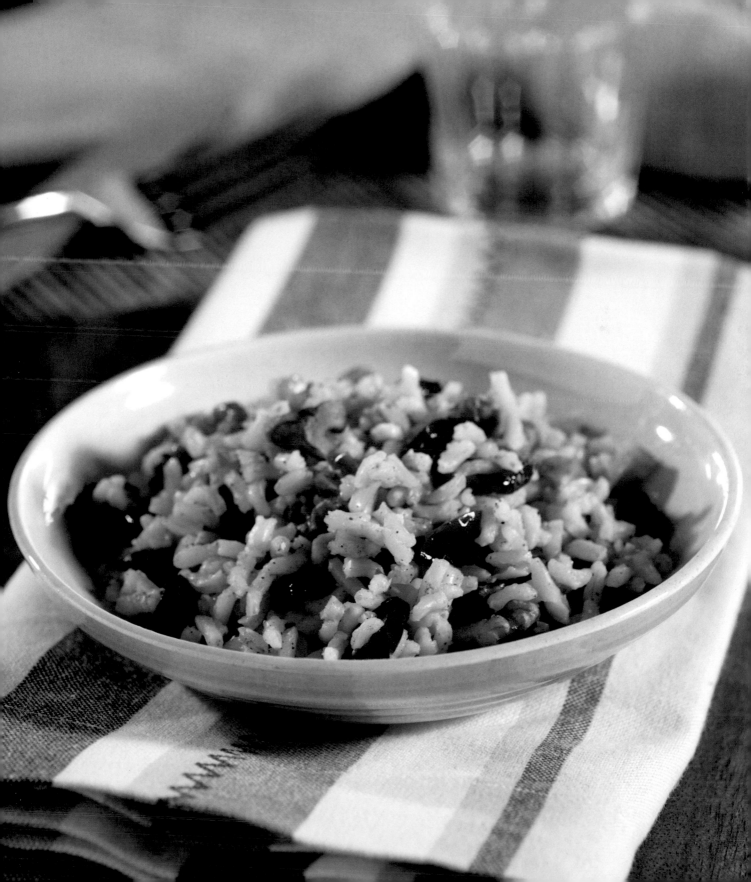

Cold Peanut Noodle & Edamame Salad

Makes 4 servings

- ½ (8-ounce) package brown rice pad thai noodles
- 3 tablespoons tamari or gluten-free soy sauce
- 2 tablespoons toasted sesame oil
- 2 tablespoons unseasoned rice vinegar
- 1 tablespoon sugar
- 1 tablespoon finely grated fresh ginger
- 1 tablespoon creamy peanut butter
- 1 tablespoon sriracha or hot chili sauce
- 2 teaspoons minced garlic
- ½ cup thawed frozen shelled edamame
- ¼ cup shredded carrots
- ¼ cup sliced green onions
- Chopped peanuts (optional)

1. Prepare noodles according to package directions for pasta. Rinse under cold water; drain. Cut noodles into 3-inch lengths. Place in large bowl; set aside.

2. Whisk tamari, oil, vinegar, sugar, ginger, peanut butter, sriracha and garlic in small bowl until smooth and well blended.

3. Pour dressing over noodles; toss gently to coat. Stir in edamame and carrots. Cover and refrigerate at least 30 minutes before serving. Top with green onions and peanuts, if desired.

Note: Brown rice pad thai noodles can be found in the Asian section of the supermarket. Regular thin rice noodles or gluten-free spaghetti may be substituted.

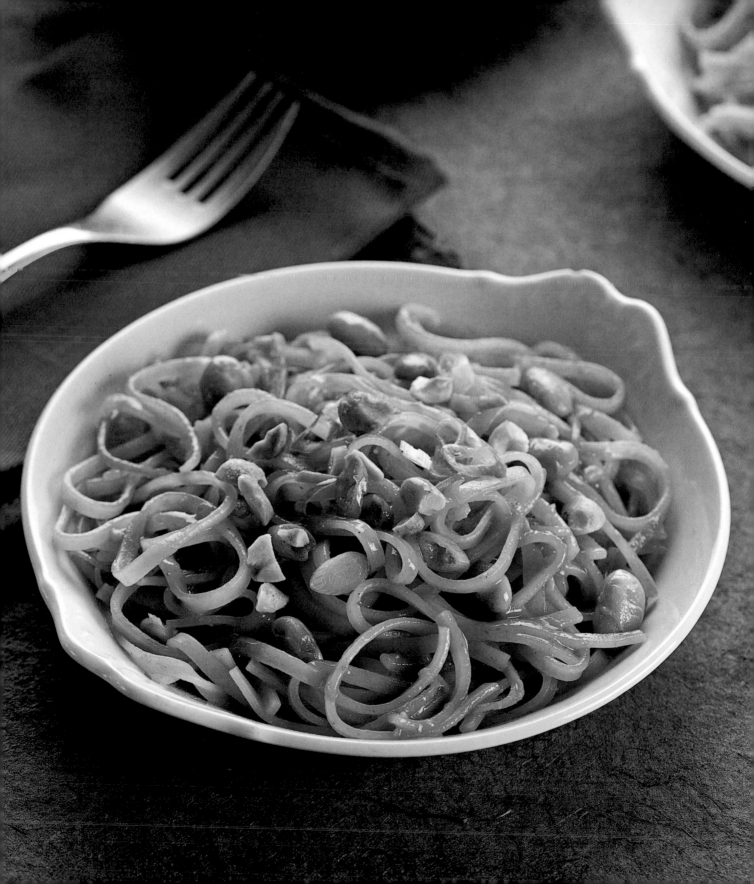

Cilantro Peanut Pesto on Soba

Makes 4 to 6 servings

1 cup packed fresh basil leaves

½ cup packed fresh cilantro leaves

¾ cup dry roasted peanuts, divided

1 jalapeño pepper, seeded

3 cloves garlic

2 teaspoons liquid aminos or tamari

1 tablespoon plus ¾ teaspoon salt, divided

½ cup peanut oil

1 package (about 12 ounces) uncooked soba noodles

Chopped fresh cilantro (optional)

1. Combine basil, ½ cup cilantro, ½ cup peanuts, jalapeño, garlic, liquid aminos and ¾ teaspoon salt in food processor; pulse until coarsely chopped. With motor running, drizzle in oil in thin steady stream; process until well blended.

2. Bring large saucepan of water to a boil. Add remaining 1 tablespoon salt; stir until dissolved. Add noodles; return to a boil. Reduce heat to low. Cook 3 minutes or until noodles are tender. Drain and rinse under cold water to cool.

3. Place noodles in medium bowl; stir in pesto. Chop remaining ¼ cup peanuts; sprinkle over noodles. Garnish with chopped cilantro.

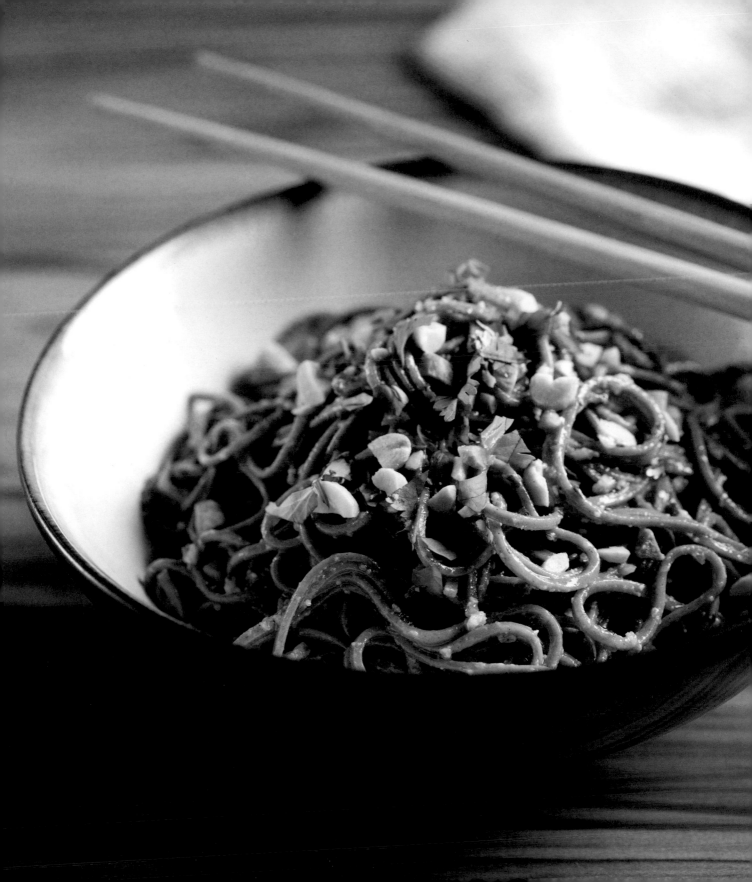

Herbed Chicken & Pasta with Spanish Olives

Makes 4 servings

4 ounces uncooked gluten-free rotini pasta

3 tablespoons olive oil, divided

1 pound boneless skinless chicken breasts, cut into bite-size pieces

½ teaspoon salt

½ teaspoon dried rosemary

¼ teaspoon dried thyme

¼ teaspoon red pepper flakes

4 cloves garlic, minced

1 cup grape tomatoes, quartered

3 ounces Spanish stuffed olives, halved lengthwise (about ½ cup)

2 tablespoons chopped fresh parsley

1½ cups packed baby spinach, coarsely chopped

1. Cook pasta in large saucepan of boiling salted water according to package directions for al dente; drain and return to saucepan.

2. Meanwhile, heat 1 tablespoon oil in large skillet over medium-high heat. Add chicken, salt, rosemary, thyme and red pepper flakes; cook and stir about 5 minutes or until chicken is no longer pink in center. Add garlic; cook and stir 30 seconds. Stir in tomatoes, olives and parsley; cook until heated through.

3. Add chicken mixture, spinach and remaining 2 tablespoons oil to pasta; toss until spinach begins to wilt.

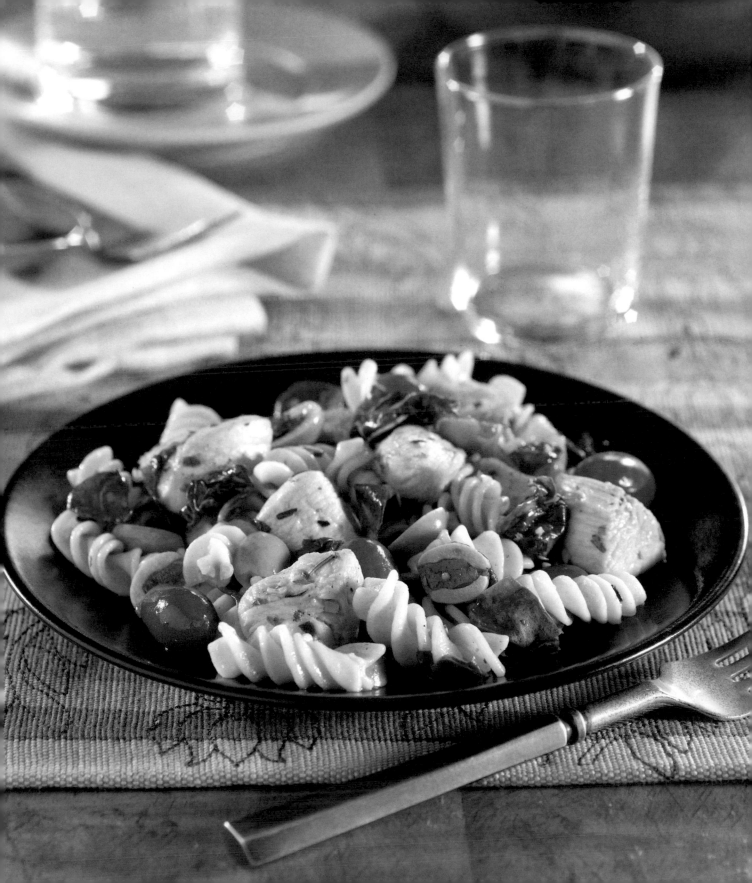

Brown Rice with Chickpeas, Spinach & Feta

Makes 4 servings

1 tablespoon olive oil

½ cup diced celery

½ cup uncooked instant brown rice

1 can (about 15 ounces) chickpeas, rinsed and drained

1 package (10 ounces) frozen chopped spinach, thawed and squeezed dry

1 teaspoon Greek or Italian seasoning

1 clove garlic, minced

½ teaspoon salt

⅛ teaspoon black pepper

2 cups water

1 tablespoon lemon juice

½ cup (2 ounces) crumbled feta cheese

1. Heat oil in large skillet over medium-high heat. Add celery; cook 4 minutes or until lightly glazed and brown in spots, stirring occasionally.

2. Stir rice, chickpeas, spinach, Greek seasoning, garlic, salt, pepper and water into skillet. Cover and bring to a boil. Reduce heat to low; simmer 12 minutes or until rice is tender. Remove from heat. Gently stir in lemon juice and cheese.

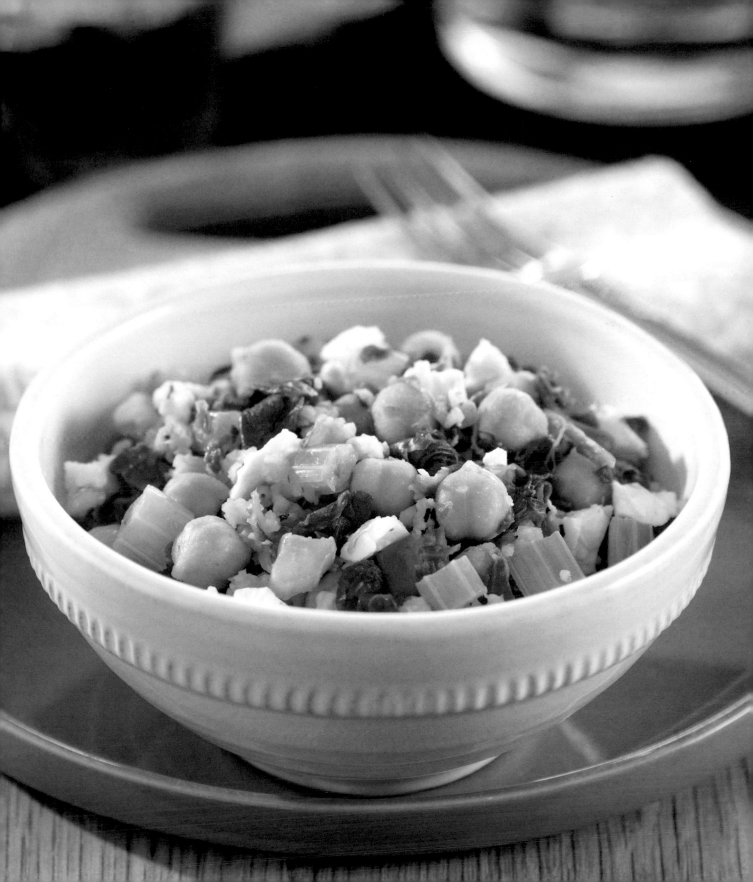

Parmesan Alfredo Pasta Bake

Makes 6 to 8 servings

- 2 tablespoons plus ½ teaspoon salt, divided
- 1 package (12 ounces) uncooked gluten-free rotini pasta
- 6 tablespoons (¾ stick) butter
- 1 clove garlic
- 1 cup whipping cream
- 1 cup milk
- 2 cups shredded Parmesan cheese, divided
- 1 cup (4 ounces) shredded mozzarella cheese
- 4 ounces mozzarella cheese, cubed
- 1 cup gluten-free panko bread crumbs
- 2 tablespoons butter, melted
- ¼ teaspoon Italian seasoning

1. Preheat oven to 400°F. Spray 3-quart baking dish with nonstick cooking spray.

2. Bring large saucepan of water to a boil; stir in 2 tablespoons salt. Add pasta; cook according to package directions until al dente. Drain pasta, reserving ½ cup cooking water. Return pasta to saucepan.

3. Meanwhile, melt 6 tablespoons butter in medium saucepan over medium heat. Add garlic and remaining ½ teaspoon salt. Stir in cream, milk and ½ cup pasta water; bring to a simmer. Remove from heat; remove and discard garlic clove. Gradually stir in 1 cup Parmesan cheese and shredded mozzarella cheese until smooth and well blended. Pour over pasta; stir gently to coat. Pour into prepared baking dish; fold in cubed mozzarella cheese.

4. Combine panko, remaining 1 cup Parmesan cheese and 2 tablespoons melted butter in medium bowl. Spread evenly over pasta mixture; sprinkle with Italian seasoning.

5. Bake 15 minutes or until topping is golden brown and pasta is heated through.

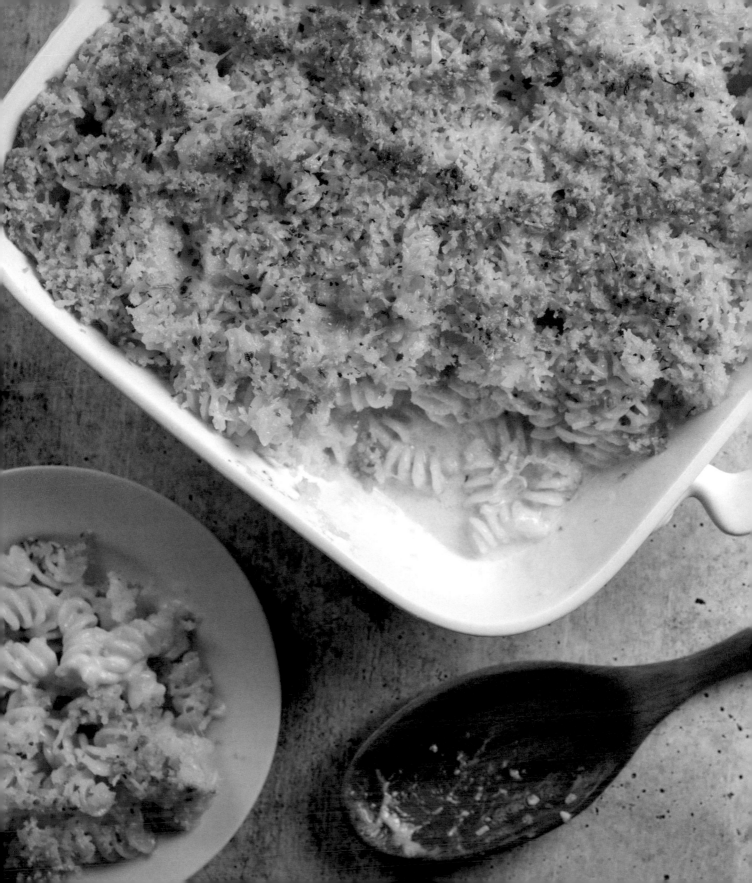

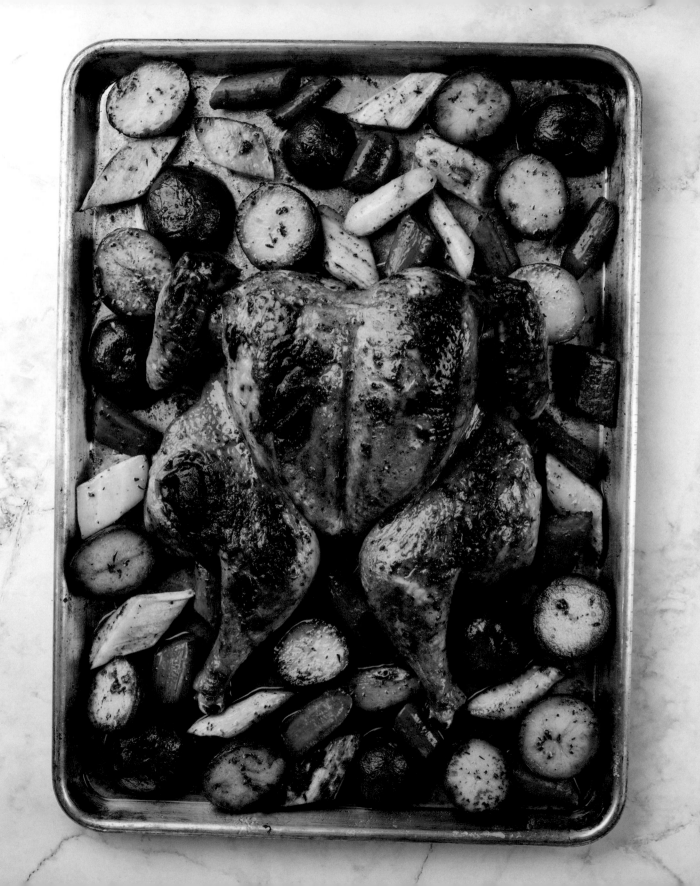

weeknight entrées

Spatchcock Chicken & Vegetables
Makes 4 servings

1 whole chicken (about 4 pounds)

6 tablespoons (¾ stick) butter, softened

2 tablespoons fresh thyme leaves

1 tablespoon honey

1 tablespoon Dijon mustard

1¼ teaspoons salt

½ teaspoon black pepper

12 ounces unpeeled small red potatoes, halved (about 12 (2-inch) potatoes)

8 ounces parsnips, cut diagonally into 1½-inch pieces (cut in half lengthwise if very thick)

8 ounces carrots, cut diagonally into 1½-inch pieces

1. Position oven rack in lower third of oven. Preheat oven to 425°F. Line baking sheet with foil, if desired.

2. To spatchcock chicken, place breast side down on cutting board. Cut along both sides of backbone with poultry shears or kitchen scissors; remove and discard backbone. Turn chicken breast side up; press down firmly on breast until it cracks to flatten chicken. Place on prepared baking sheet.

3. Combine butter, thyme, honey, mustard, salt and pepper in small microwavable bowl; mix well. Rub 1 tablespoon mixture under skin of chicken breast. Rub 1 tablespoon mixture all over chicken skin.

4. Combine potatoes, parsnips and carrots in large bowl. Melt remaining butter mixture in microwave; pour over vegetables and toss to coat. Arrange vegetables around chicken on baking sheet.

5. Roast 50 to 60 minutes or until chicken is cooked through (165°F), covering chicken loosely with foil after 30 minutes if skin is turning too dark. Remove chicken to clean cutting board; tent with foil and let stand 10 minutes before slicing. Serve with vegetables.

Mongolian Beef

Makes 4 servings

1¼ **pounds beef flank steak**

¼ **cup cornstarch**

3 **tablespoons vegetable oil, divided**

3 **cloves garlic, minced**

2 **teaspoons grated fresh ginger**

½ **cup water**

½ **cup tamari or gluten-free soy sauce**

⅓ **cup packed dark brown sugar**

Pinch red pepper flakes

2 **green onions, diagonally sliced into 1-inch pieces**

Hot cooked rice (optional)

1. Cut flank steak in half lengthwise, then cut crosswise (against the grain) into ¼-inch slices. Combine beef and cornstarch in medium bowl; toss to coat.

2. Heat 1 tablespoon oil in large skillet or wok over high heat. Add half of beef in single layer (do not crowd); cook 1 to 2 minutes per side or until browned. Remove to clean bowl. Repeat with remaining beef and 1 tablespoon oil.

3. Heat remaining 1 tablespoon oil in same skillet over medium heat. Add garlic and ginger; cook and stir 30 seconds. Add water, tamari, brown sugar and red pepper flakes; bring to a boil, stirring until well blended. Cook 8 minutes or until slightly thickened, stirring occasionally.

4. Return beef to skillet; cook 2 to 3 minutes or until sauce thickens and beef is heated through. Stir in green onions. Serve with rice, if desired.

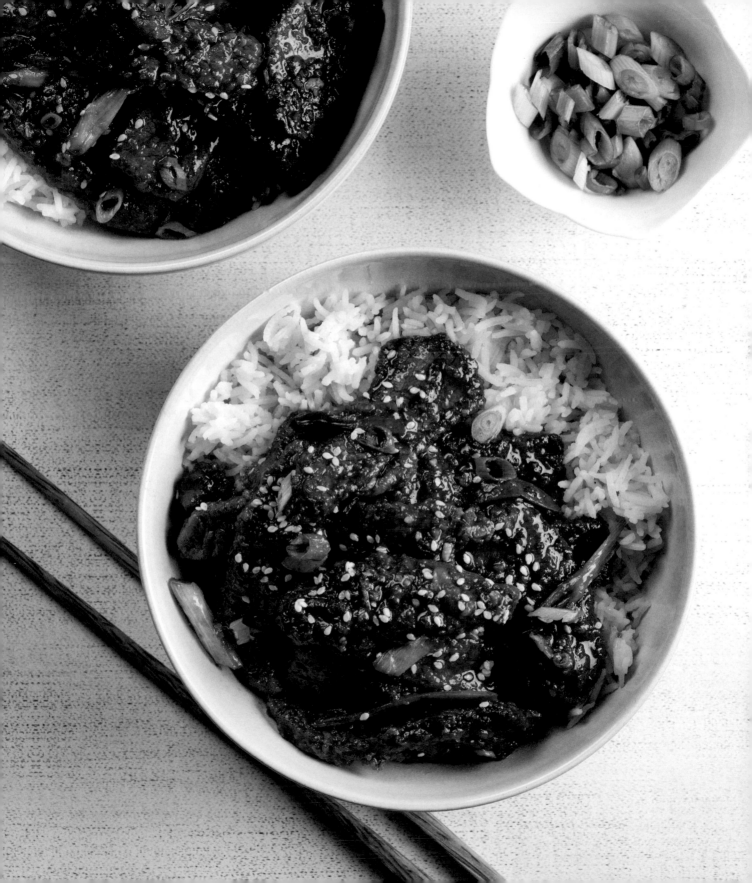

Spicy Tuna Sushi Bowl

Makes 2 servings

2 tablespoons mayonnaise

1 teaspoon sriracha or hot chile sauce

3 teaspoons unseasoned rice wine vinegar, divided

1 tuna steak (about 6 ounces)

1 cup hot cooked brown rice

½ cup diced cucumber

½ ripe avocado, sliced

Black sesame seeds (optional)

1. Whisk mayonnaise, sriracha and 1 teaspoon vinegar in small bowl. Rub tuna evenly with half of sauce. Marinate 10 minutes.

2. Meanwhile, stir remaining 2 teaspoons vinegar into rice; set aside.

3. Heat small nonstick skillet over medium-high heat. Cook tuna 2 minutes per side for medium rare or until desired doneness. Slice tuna.

4. Divide rice, cucumber, avocado and tuna slices between two bowls. Sprinkle with sesame seeds, if desired. Serve with remaining sauce.

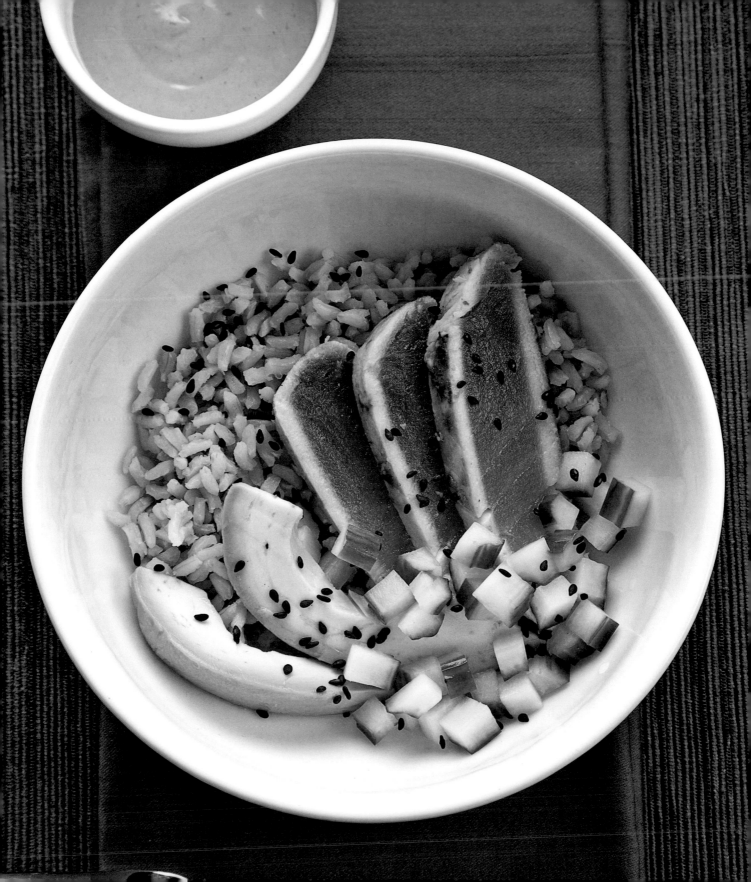

Beef & Turkey Meat Loaf

Makes 4 servings

¾ **pound ground beef**

¾ **pound ground turkey**

½ **cup grated carrot**

⅓ **cup finely chopped onion**

⅓ **cup crushed gluten-free corn or rice cereal squares**

⅓ **cup plus 2 tablespoons chili sauce, divided**

1 **egg, beaten**

¾ **teaspoon salt**

½ **teaspoon black pepper**

1. Preheat oven to 350°F. Spray 13×9-inch pan with nonstick cooking spray.

2. Combine beef, turkey, carrot, onion, cereal, ⅓ cup chili sauce, egg, salt and pepper in large bowl; mix well.

3. Shape into 8-inch-long loaf; place in prepared pan. Spread remaining 2 tablespoons chili sauce evenly over top of meat loaf.

4. Bake 1 hour and 15 minutes or until cooked through (165°F). Cool in pan 10 minutes; cut into slices to serve.

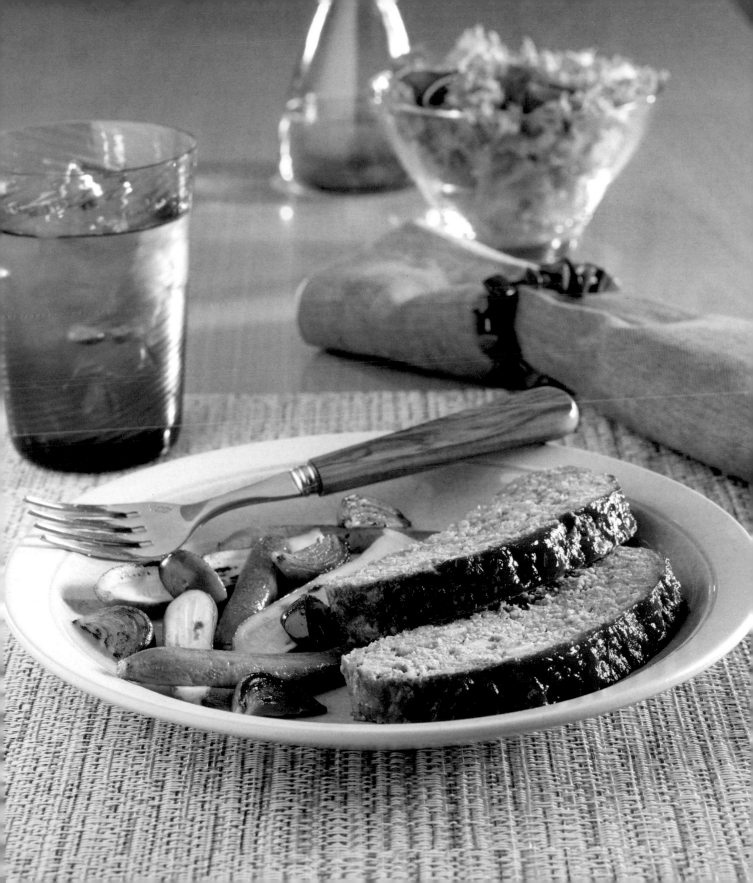

Spaghetti Squash Alfredo

Makes 4 servings

¼ cup (½ stick) butter

1 teaspoon minced garlic

4 cups cooked spaghetti squash (see Tip)

½ teaspoon salt

½ teaspoon black pepper

1 cup whipping cream

½ cup grated Parmesan cheese, plus additional for garnish

1 tablespoon olive oil

12 ounces (about 2 cups) frozen cooked shrimp, thawed

Chopped fresh basil (optional)

1. Melt butter in large nonstick skillet over medium-high heat. Add garlic; cook 30 seconds. Add squash, salt and pepper; cook and stir 2 to 3 minutes or until heated through. Add cream; cook and stir 3 minutes or until sauce begins to thicken. Reduce heat to low. Stir in ½ cup cheese; cook 2 minutes or until cheese is melted, stirring constantly. Cover and keep warm.

2. Meanwhile, heat oil in large nonstick skillet over high heat. Add shrimp; cook and stir until heated through.

3. Divide squash among four bowls. Top with shrimp and garnish with additional cheese and basil.

Tip: Two medium spaghetti squash (3 to 3½ pounds) will yield about 4 cups cooked squash. To cook squash easily and quickly, pierce each squash to the center with a knife in two places. Place squash on a microwavable plate and microwave on HIGH 20 minutes. (If the microwave does not have an automatic turntable, turn squash three times during cooking.) Let stand 10 minutes. Cut off stem end and discard. Slice in half lengthwise. Scoop out seeds and center membranes and discard. Using a fork, pull squash into strands and drain in colander.

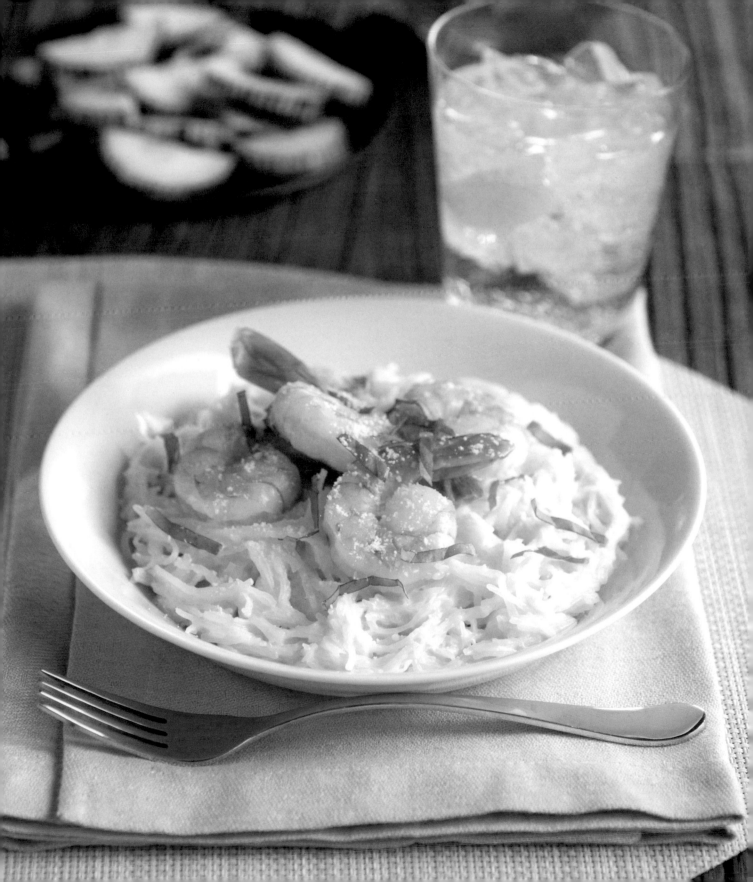

Southwest Chicken Burgers with Avocado Salad

Makes 6 servings

1 cup finely diced yellow or red bell pepper, divided

½ cup finely diced red onion, divided

1 egg white

1½ teaspoons chili powder, divided

1¼ teaspoons salt, divided

¼ teaspoon black pepper

20 ounces ground chicken

2 medium avocados, diced

¾ cup finely diced cucumber

Juice of 1 lime

2 tablespoons vegetable oil

6 tablespoons shredded Cheddar cheese

1. Combine ½ cup bell pepper, ¼ cup onion, egg white, 1 teaspoon chili powder, 1 teaspoon salt and black pepper in large bowl. Add chicken; mix well. Shape mixture into six patties. Place on cutting board; cover and refrigerate 15 minutes.

2. Combine avocados, cucumber, lime juice, remaining ½ cup bell pepper, ¼ cup onion, ½ teaspoon chili powder and ¼ teaspoon salt in medium bowl.

3. Heat 1 tablespoon oil in large skillet over medium heat. Add half of burgers; cook 5 minutes. Turn and top each burger with 1 tablespoon cheese. Cook 5 minutes or until no longer pink in center. Repeat with remaining oil, burgers and cheese.

4. Divide avocado salad among six plates; top with burgers.

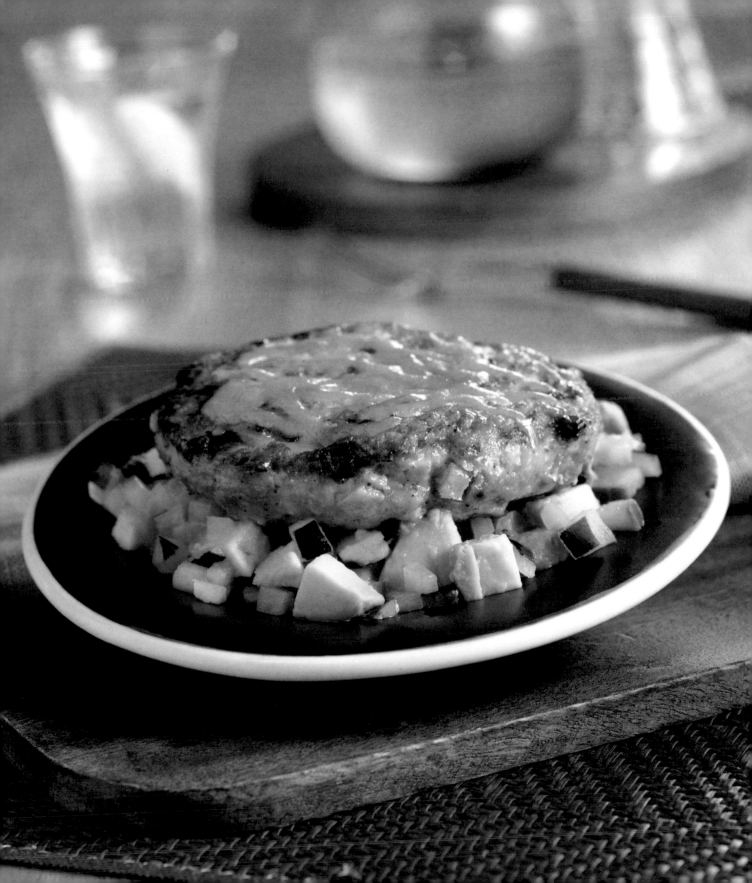

Pan-Fried Gnocchi Skillet

Makes 6 servings

1 pound baking potatoes (about 2 medium), cut into 1-inch pieces

½ cup grated Parmesan cheese, divided

3 tablespoons rice flour, plus additional for work surface

1 egg

1 egg white

½ teaspoon salt

1 tablespoon olive oil

¾ pound bulk hot Italian sausage, casings removed

2 large zucchini, diced

1 cup sliced cremini mushrooms

1 can (about 14 ounces) diced tomatoes with basil, garlic and oregano, drained

1. Place potatoes in large microwavable bowl. Cover; microwave on HIGH 8 to 10 minutes or until very tender. Cool 10 minutes. Peel potatoes.

2. Meanwhile, combine cheese, 3 tablespoons rice flour, egg, egg white and salt in medium bowl; mix well. Mash or press potatoes through ricer into cheese mixture.

3. Heavily dust cutting board or work surface with rice flour. Working in batches, scoop portions of dough onto board and roll into ½-inch-thick rope using rice-floured hands. Cut each rope into ¾-inch pieces. Cover unrolled dough with damp paper towel to keep from drying out.

4. Heat oil in large nonstick skillet over medium heat. Working in batches, add gnocchi in single layer and cook 5 minutes per side until lightly browned and heated through, turning once. Remove from skillet; keep warm.

5. Cook sausage in same skillet over medium-high heat 8 to 10 minutes or until no longer pink, stirring to break up meat. Add zucchini and mushrooms; cook and stir 3 to 5 minutes or until crisp-tender. Add tomatoes; cook until heated through. Return gnocchi to skillet; gently toss.

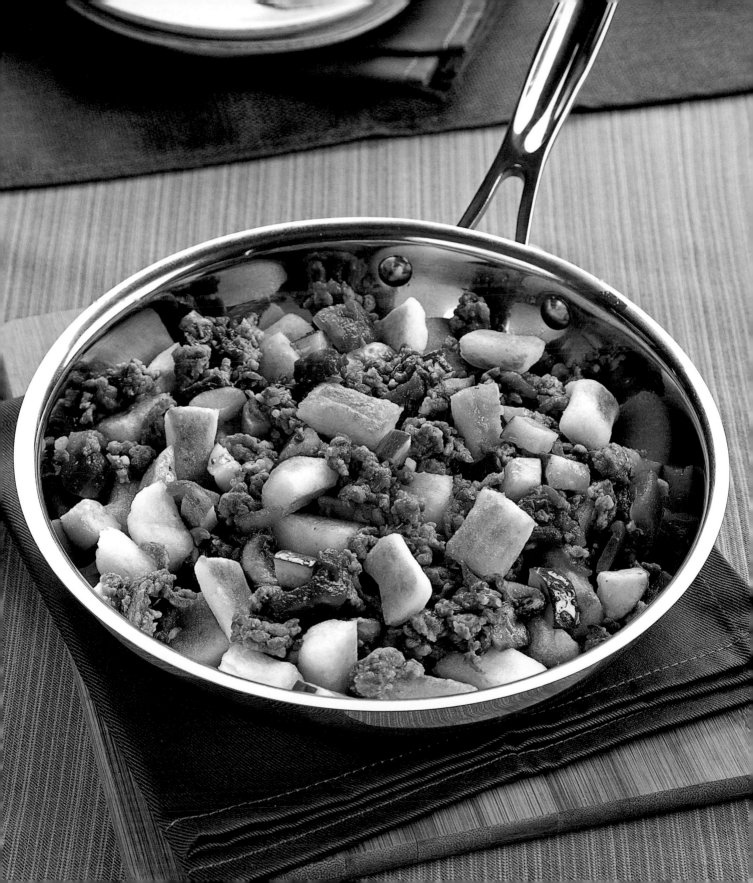

Herbed Pork with Potatoes & Green Beans

Makes 4 servings

2 tablespoons chopped fresh thyme

2 tablespoons chopped fresh rosemary

2 cloves garlic, minced

2 teaspoons salt

¾ teaspoon black pepper

¼ cup olive oil

1½ pounds fingerling potatoes (about 18 potatoes), cut in half lengthwise

1 pound green beans

2 pork tenderloins (about 12 ounces each)

1. Preheat oven to 450°F. Combine thyme, rosemary, garlic, salt and pepper in small bowl. Stir in oil until well blended.

2. Place potatoes in medium bowl. Drizzle with one third of oil mixture, toss to coat. Arrange potatoes, cut sides down, in rows covering two thirds of large baking sheet. (Potatoes should be in single layer; do not overlap.) Leave remaining one third of baking sheet empty.

3. Roast potatoes 10 minutes while preparing beans and pork. Trim green beans; place in same bowl used for potatoes. Drizzle with one third of oil mixture; toss to coat. When potatoes have roasted 10 minutes, remove baking sheet from oven. Arrange green beans on empty third of baking sheet. Brush all sides of pork with remaining oil mixture; place on top of green beans.

4. Roast 20 to 25 minutes or until pork is 145°F. Transfer pork to large cutting board. Tent with foil; let stand 10 minutes.

5. Stir vegetables; return to oven. Roast 10 minutes or until golden brown. Slice pork; serve with vegetables.

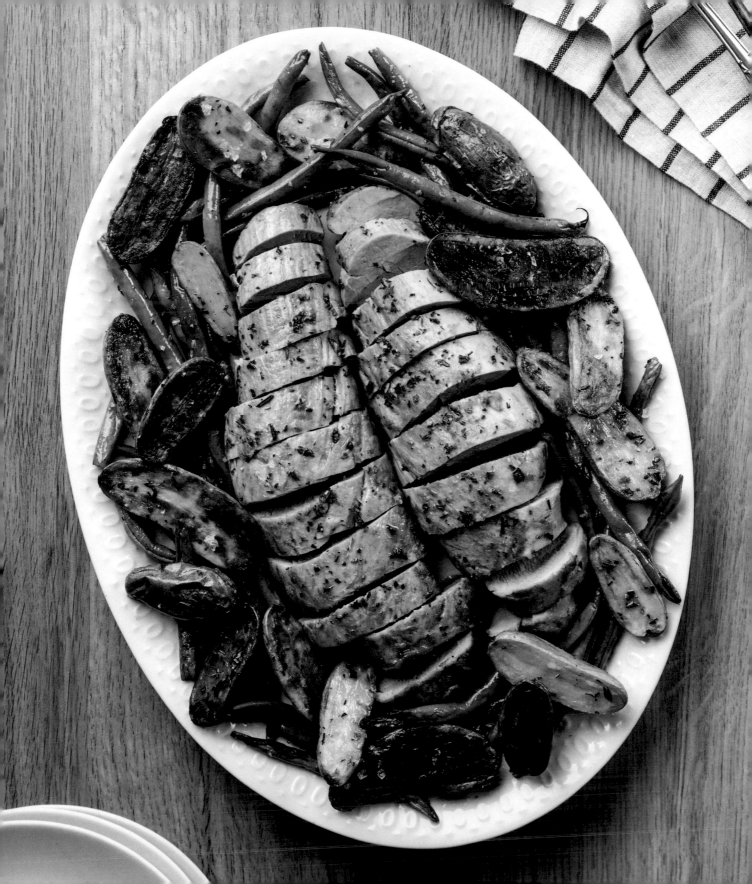

Peri-Peri Chicken

Makes 4 servings

- 1 small red onion, coarsely chopped
- 1 roasted red pepper (about 3 ounces)
- ¼ cup olive oil
- ¼ cup lemon juice
- 2 tablespoons white vinegar
- 4 cloves garlic, minced
- 1 tablespoon smoked paprika
- 1½ teaspoons salt
- 1½ teaspoons red pepper flakes
- 1 teaspoon dried oregano
- ½ teaspoon black pepper
- 1 cut-up whole chicken (3 to 4 pounds)

1. Combine onion, roasted pepper, oil, lemon juice, vinegar, garlic, paprika, salt, red pepper flakes, oregano and black pepper in blender or food processor; blend until smooth. Remove half of marinade to small bowl; cover and refrigerate until ready to use.

2. Use sharp knife to make several slashes in each piece of chicken (about ¼ inch deep). Place chicken in large resealable food storage bag. Pour remaining marinade over chicken; seal bag and turn to coat, massaging marinade into chicken. Marinate in refrigerator at least 4 hours or overnight, turning occasionally.

3. Remove chicken from refrigerator about 30 minutes before cooking. Preheat oven to 400°F.* Line baking sheet with foil. Arrange chicken on baking sheet.

4. Bake about 45 minutes or until chicken is cooked through (165°F), brushing with some of reserved marinade every 15 minutes. Serve with remaining marinade, if desired.

For a smokier flavor, grill chicken over medium heat 30 to 40 minutes or until cooked through (165°F).

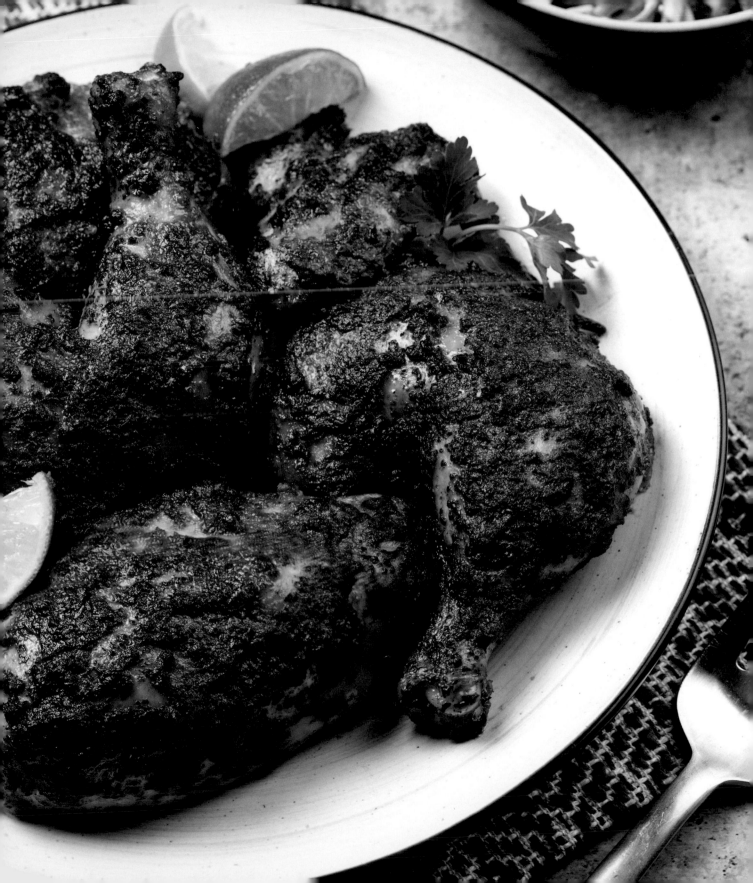

Cauliflower Parmesan

Makes 4 servings

2   heads cauliflower (about
    2 pounds each)

1   tablespoon plus 2 teaspoons
    olive oil, divided

2   teaspoons salt, divided

    Black pepper

3   tablespoons butter

1   medium onion, chopped

2   cloves garlic, minced

1   teaspoon dried oregano

½   teaspoon dried basil

¼   teaspoon red pepper flakes
    (optional)

1   can (28 ounces) crushed
    tomatoes

1   can (about 14 ounces) diced
    tomatoes

⅓   cup shredded Parmesan cheese

4   slices fresh mozzarella cheese
    (1 ounce each)

    Shredded fresh basil (optional)

1. Preheat oven to 425°F. Turn cauliflower stem side up on cutting board. Trim away leaves, leaving stem intact. Slice through stem into 2 or 3 slices. Trim off excess florets from two end slices, creating flat "steaks." Repeat with remaining cauliflower; reserve extra cauliflower for another use.

2. Grease large baking sheet with 2 teaspoons oil. Place 4 steaks on baking sheet. Brush remaining 1 tablespoon oil over cauliflower; sprinkle with 1 teaspoon salt and season with pepper. Bake 25 minutes or until fork-tender and well browned.

3. Meanwhile for sauce, melt butter in large saucepan over medium-high heat. Add onion; cook and stir 5 minutes or until softened. Add garlic, remaining 1 teaspoon salt, oregano, basil and red pepper flakes, if desired; cook and stir 1 minute. Add tomatoes; mix well. Bring to a simmer. Reduce heat to medium; partially cover and cook 20 minutes.

4. *Reduce oven temperature to 375°F.* Spray 13×9-inch baking pan with nonstick cooking spray. Spread 2 cups sauce in pan. Using large spatula, carefully transfer cauliflower to baking pan. Spread ¼ cup sauce over each steak; sprinkle evenly with Parmesan cheese. Top each with slice of mozzarella cheese.

5. Bake 12 to 15 minutes or until cheese is melted and browned in spots and sauce is bubbly. Garnish with fresh basil.

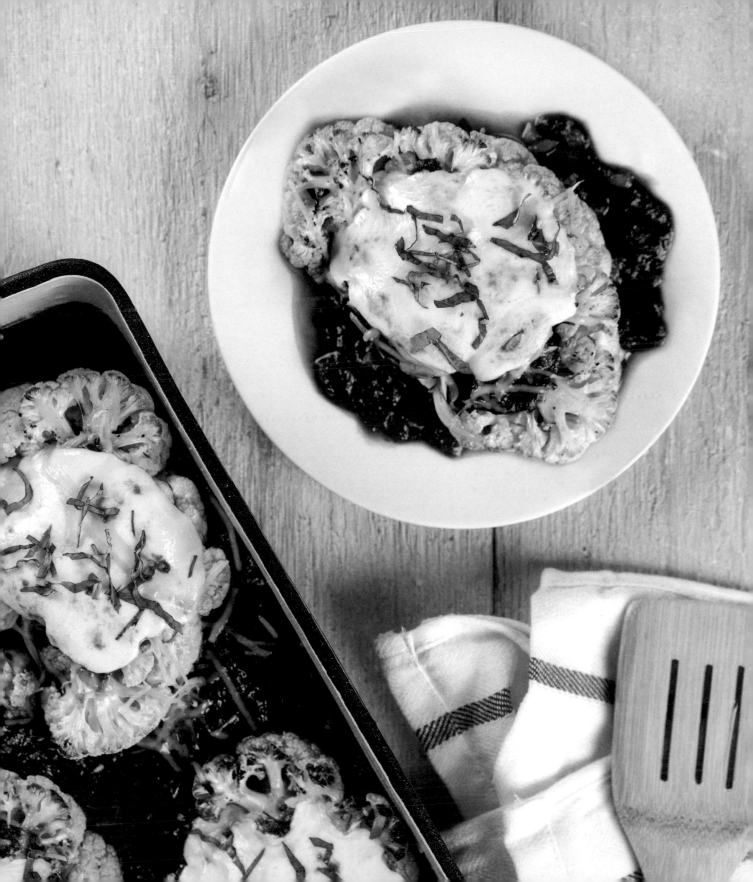

Flourless Fried Chicken Tenders

Makes 4 servings

1½ cups chickpea flour

1½ teaspoons Italian seasoning

1 teaspoon salt

½ teaspoon black pepper

⅛ teaspoon ground red pepper

¾ cup plus 2 to 4 tablespoons water

Curry Mayo Dipping Sauce (recipe follows, optional)

Vegetable oil

1 pound chicken tenders, cut in half if large

1. Sift chickpea flour into medium bowl. Stir in Italian seasoning, salt, black pepper and red pepper. Gradually whisk in ¾ cup water until smooth. Whisk in additional water by tablespoons until batter is consistency of heavy cream.

2. Prepare Curry Mayo Dipping Sauce, if desired. Pour 1 inch of oil in large heavy skillet or Dutch oven. Heat over medium-high heat until oil registers 350°F on deep-fry thermometer or drop of batter placed in oil sizzles.

3. Pat chicken pieces dry. Dip chicken into batter with tongs; let excess drip back into bowl. Slide chicken gently into oil in batches. (Do not crowd pan.) Fry 2 to 3 minutes per side or until slightly browned and chicken is cooked through.

4. Drain chicken on paper towels. Serve warm with dipping sauce.

Curry Mayo Dipping Sauce: Combine ½ cup mayonnaise, ¼ cup sour cream and ½ teaspoon curry powder in small bowl. Stir in 2 tablespoons minced fresh cilantro.

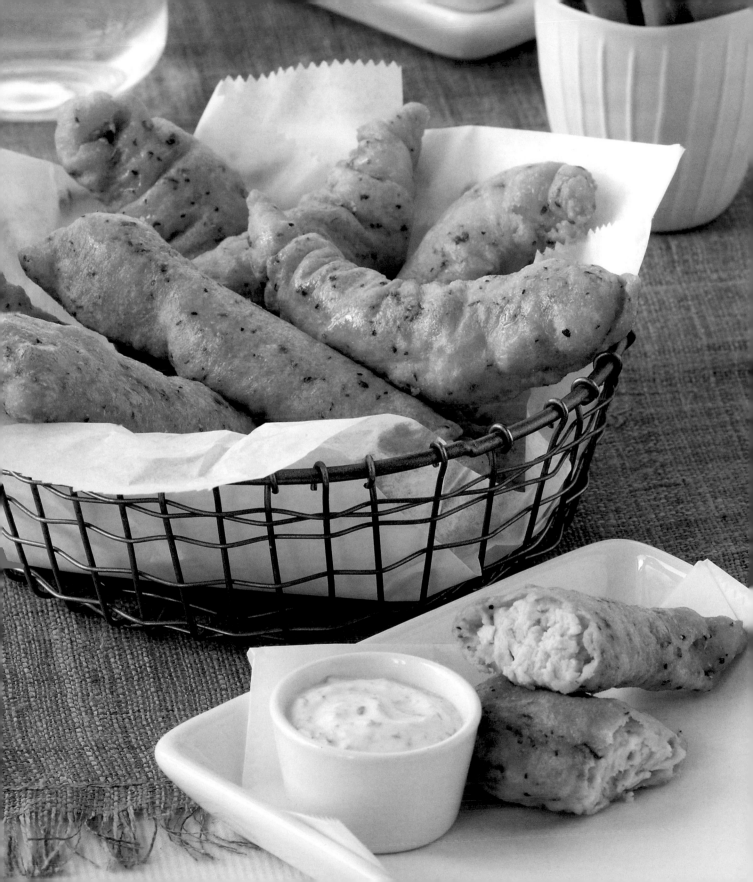

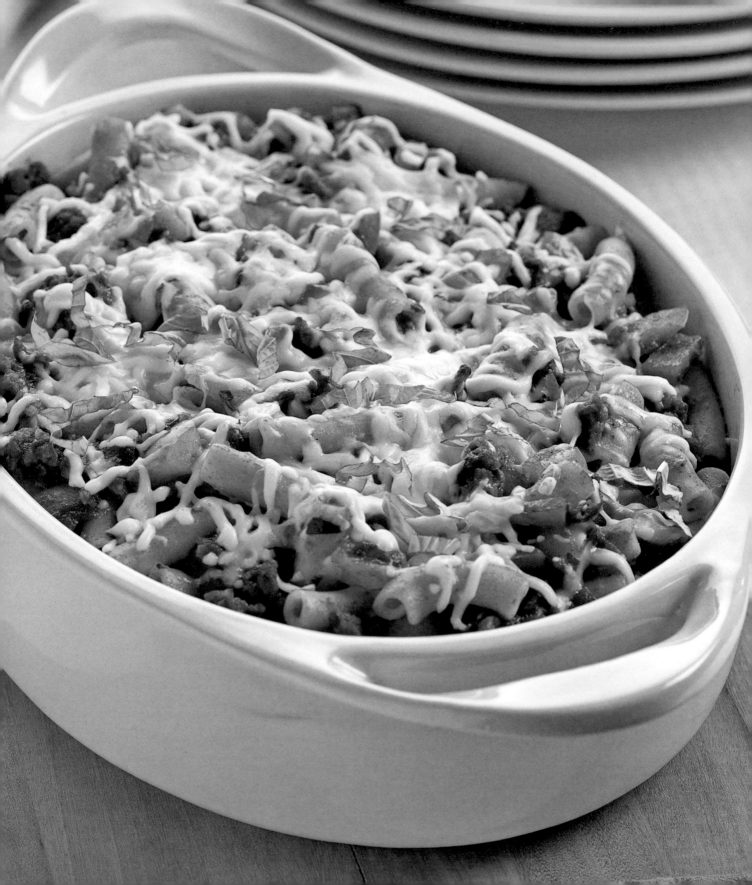

hearty casseroles

Baked Penne with Sausage & Peppers

Makes 8 servings

- 8 ounces uncooked gluten-free penne pasta
- 1 tablespoon olive oil
- 1 pound hot or mild Italian sausage, casings removed
- 1 large yellow bell pepper, cut into ½-inch pieces
- 1 large green bell pepper, cut into ½-inch pieces
- 1 jar (24 ounces) tomato-basil marinara sauce
- 2 cups (8 ounces) shredded mozzarella cheese, divided
- Chopped fresh basil (optional)

1. Preheat oven to 350°F.

2. Cook pasta in large saucepan of salted boiling water according to package directions for al dente. Drain.

3. Meanwhile, heat oil in large nonstick skillet over medium heat. Crumble sausage into skillet; cook 5 minutes or until browned, stirring to break up meat. Add bell peppers; cook 5 to 7 minutes or until sausage is no longer pink and bell peppers are crisp-tender. Drain fat.

4. Add marinara sauce to skillet; cook 3 minutes or until heated through. Stir in penne.

5. Spread half of penne mixture in 2-quart baking dish. Top with 1 cup cheese. Layer with remaining penne mixture and 1 cup cheese.

6. Bake 25 to 30 minutes or until heated through and cheese is melted. Garnish with basil.

Chicken Stew with Polenta Dumplings

Makes 6 servings

2 pounds boneless skinless chicken thighs

Salt and black pepper

4 tablespoons olive oil, divided

2 medium eggplants, chopped

4 medium onions, chopped

4 tomatoes, seeded and diced

1 cup chicken broth

⅓ cup pitted black olives, sliced

1 tablespoon chopped fresh thyme *or* 1 teaspoon dried thyme

1 tablespoon red wine vinegar

Polenta Dumplings

3½ cups chicken broth

1 cup polenta or yellow cornmeal

½ cup grated Parmesan cheese

¼ cup chopped fresh parsley

1 egg, beaten

2 tablespoons butter

½ teaspoon salt

1. Preheat oven to 350°F.

2. Season chicken all over with salt and pepper. Heat 1 tablespoon oil in Dutch oven over medium-high heat. Cook chicken in batches 5 minutes or until browned on both sides, turning once. Transfer to plate.

3. Heat remaining 3 tablespoons oil in same Dutch oven; add eggplants, onions and tomatoes. Reduce heat to medium; cook and stir 5 minutes. Return chicken to Dutch oven. Stir in 1 cup broth, olives, thyme and vinegar. Bring to a boil. Cover and bake 1 hour.

4. Meanwhile for dumplings, bring 3½ cups broth to a boil in medium saucepan over medium-high heat. Gradually whisk in polenta. Reduce heat to medium-low; simmer 15 minutes or until thickened, stirring constantly. Remove from heat; stir in cheese, parsley, egg, butter and ½ teaspoon salt.

5. Top stew with rounded tablespoonfuls dumpling mixture. Bake, uncovered, 20 minutes or until dumplings are cooked through.

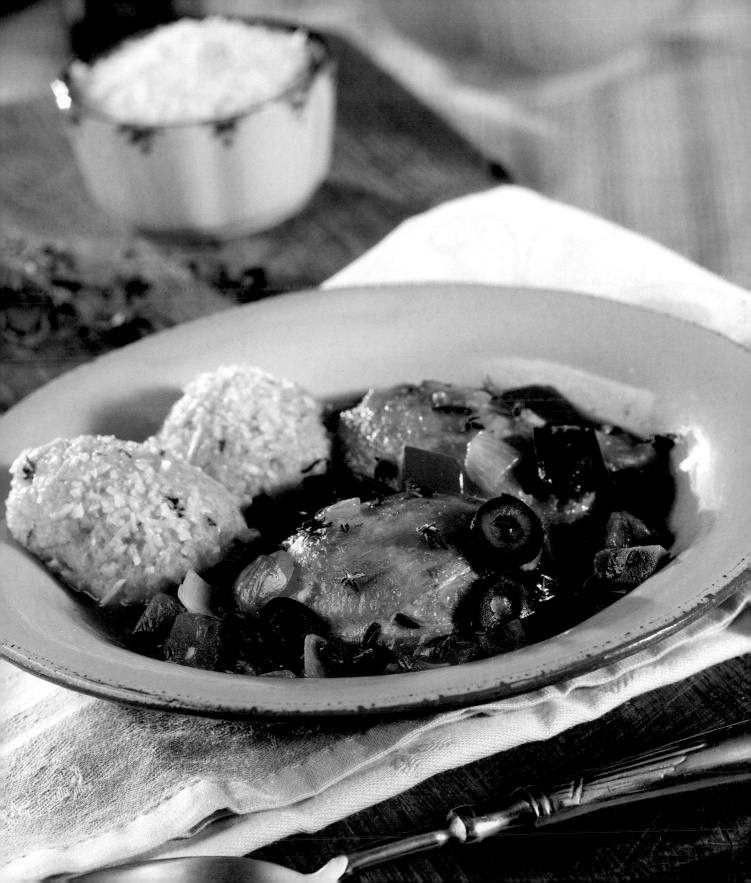

Farm-Style Casserole

Makes 4 to 6 servings

1 tablespoon canola oil

1 onion, chopped

1 clove garlic, minced

1 pound ground beef

1 can (about 14 ounces) diced tomatoes

1 cup frozen corn

1 cup frozen baby lima beans

1 teaspoon salt

½ teaspoon dried oregano

¼ teaspoon black pepper

2 cups cooked gluten-free macaroni or other shape

1 cup crushed tortilla chips

1. Preheat oven to 350°F. Heat oil in large nonstick skillet over medium heat. Add onion and garlic; cook and stir 5 to 6 minutes or until onion is softened. Add beef; cook 6 to 8 minutes or until browned, stirring to break up meat. Drain fat.

2. Stir in tomatoes, corn, lima beans, salt, oregano and pepper. Increase heat to high; cook and stir 5 minutes or until all liquid is evaporated. Stir in macaroni. Spoon mixture into 9-inch square baking dish. Sprinkle with tortilla chips.

3. Bake 20 minutes or until heated through.

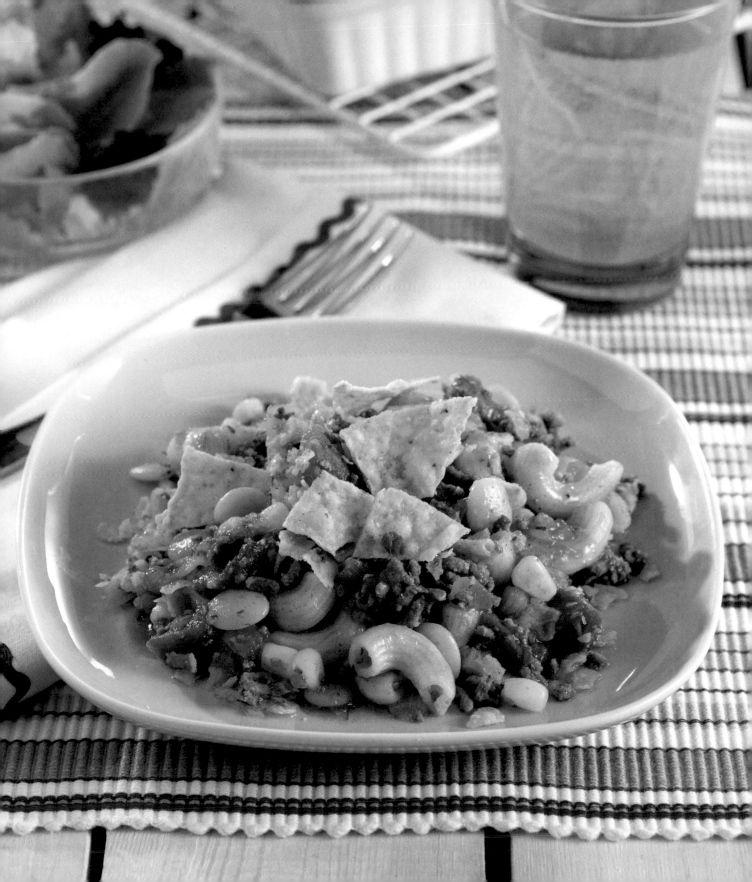

Frankfurters with Rice & Red Beans

Makes 6 servings

1   tablespoon vegetable oil

1   onion, chopped

½   green bell pepper, chopped

2   cloves garlic, minced

1   can (about 15 ounces) red kidney beans, rinsed and drained

1   can (about 15 ounces) Great Northern beans, rinsed and drained

½   pound beef frankfurters, cut into ¼-inch-thick pieces

1   cup uncooked instant brown rice

1   cup vegetable broth

¼   cup packed brown sugar

¼   cup ketchup

3   tablespoons dark molasses

1   tablespoon Dijon mustard

1. Preheat oven to 350°F. Spray 13×9-inch baking dish with nonstick cooking spray.

2. Heat oil in large saucepan over medium-high heat. Add onion, bell pepper and garlic; cook and stir 5 minutes or until vegetables are softened.

3. Add beans, frankfurters, rice, broth, brown sugar, ketchup, molasses and mustard to saucepan; gently stir until blended. Transfer to prepared baking dish.

4. Cover and bake 30 minutes or until rice is tender.

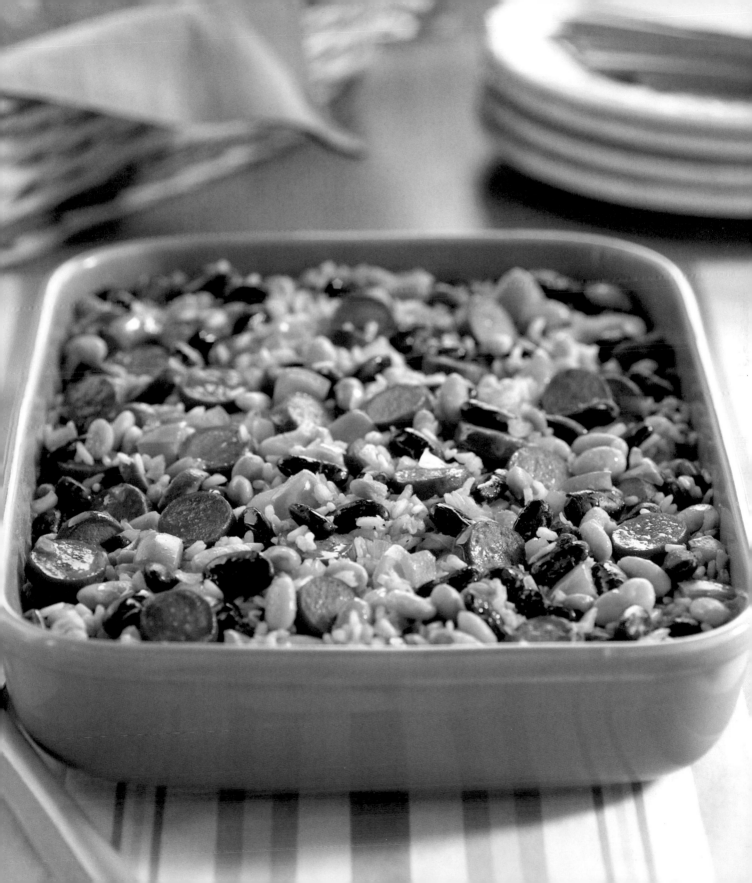

Spinach, Artichoke & Chicken Casserole

Makes 4 servings

2 cups frozen chopped spinach, thawed and squeezed dry

8 canned artichoke hearts, drained and chopped

1 cup chopped onion

¾ cup grated Parmesan cheese, divided

½ cup mayonnaise

1 teaspoon minced garlic

¼ teaspoon black pepper

2 cups chopped cooked chicken

1. Preheat oven to 375°F. Spray 2-quart baking dish with nonstick cooking spray.

2. Combine spinach, artichoke hearts, onion, ¼ cup cheese, mayonnaise, garlic and pepper in medium bowl. Place chicken in prepared baking dish; top evenly with spinach mixture. Top with remaining ½ cup cheese.

3. Bake 30 minutes or until casserole is heated through and cheese is browned.

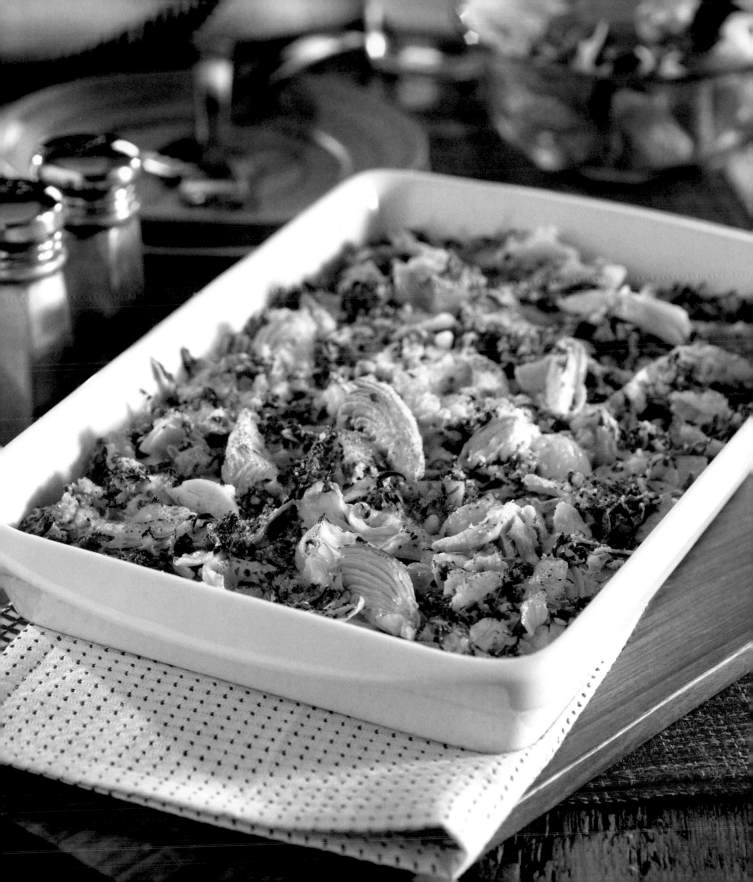

Cheesy Spinach Casserole

Makes 6 servings

1 pound baby spinach

4 slices bacon, chopped

1 small onion, chopped

1 cup sliced mushrooms

¼ cup chopped red bell pepper

3 cloves garlic, minced

1½ teaspoons minced canned chipotle peppers in adobo sauce

1 teaspoon seasoned salt

8 ounces pasteurized process cheese product, cut into pieces

½ (8-ounce) package cream cheese, cut into pieces

1 cup thawed frozen corn

½ cup (2 ounces) shredded Monterey Jack and Cheddar cheese blend

1. Preheat oven to 350°F. Spray 1-quart baking dish with nonstick cooking spray.

2. Bring large saucepan of water to a boil over high heat. Add spinach; cook 1 minute. Drain and transfer to bowl of ice water to stop cooking. Drain and squeeze spinach dry; set aside. Wipe out saucepan with paper towel.

3. Cook bacon in same saucepan over medium-high heat until almost crisp, stirring frequently. Drain off all but 1 tablespoon drippings. Add onion to saucepan; cook and stir 3 minutes or until softened. Add mushrooms and bell pepper; cook and stir 5 minutes or until vegetables are tender. Add garlic, chipotle peppers and seasoned salt; cook and stir 1 minute.

4. Add cheese product and cream cheese to saucepan; cook over medium heat until melted, stirring frequently. Add spinach and corn; cook and stir 3 minutes. Transfer to prepared baking dish; sprinkle with shredded cheese.

5. Bake 20 to 25 minutes or until cheese is melted and casserole is bubbly. If desired, broil 1 to 2 minutes to brown top of casserole.

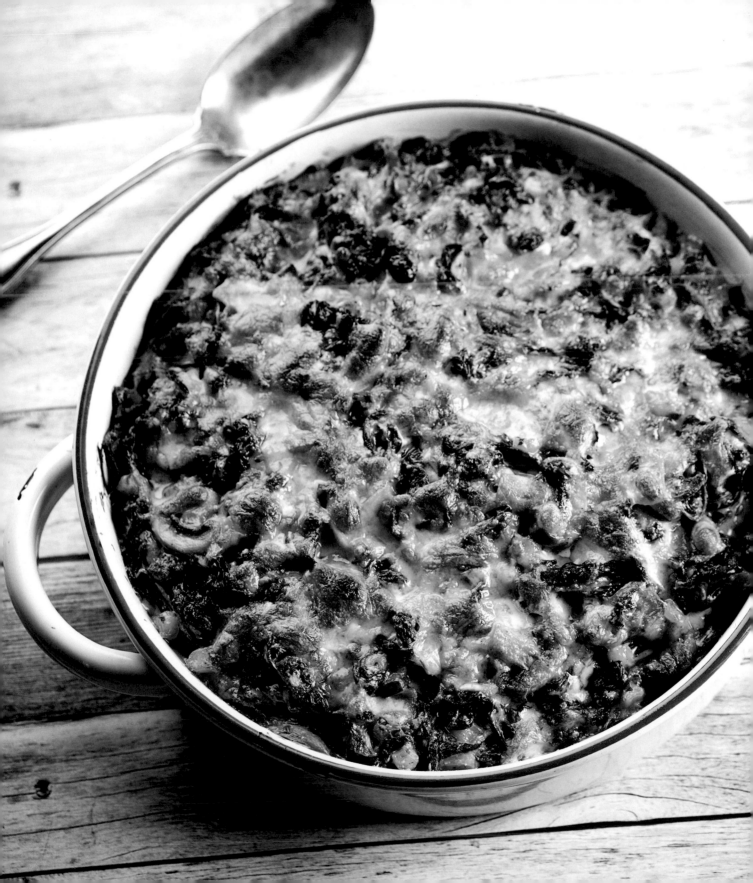

Polenta Lasagna

Makes 6 servings

4 cups water

1½ cups yellow cornmeal

4 teaspoons finely chopped fresh marjoram or oregano

1½ teaspoon salt, divided

1 teaspoon olive oil

1 pound mushrooms, sliced

1 cup chopped leeks

1 clove garlic, minced

2 tablespoons chopped fresh basil

1 tablespoon chopped fresh oregano

⅛ teaspoon black pepper

1 cup marinara sauce

½ cup (2 ounces) shredded mozzarella cheese

4 tablespoons grated Parmesan cheese

1. Bring water to a boil in medium saucepan over high heat. Slowly add cornmeal, stirring constantly. Reduce heat to low; stir in marjoram and 1 teaspoon salt. Simmer 15 to 20 minutes or until polenta thickens and pulls away from side of pan. Spread in ungreased 13×9-inch baking pan. Cover and refrigerate about 1 hour or until firm.*

2. Preheat oven to 350°F. Spray 11×7-inch baking dish with nonstick cooking spray.

3. Heat oil in large nonstick skillet over medium heat. Add mushrooms, leeks and garlic; cook and stir 5 minutes or until leeks are crisp-tender. Stir in basil, oregano, pepper and remaining ½ teaspoon salt.

4. Cut cold polenta into 12 (3½-inch) squares; arrange 6 squares in prepared baking dish. Spread with ½ cup marinara sauce, half of vegetable mixture, ¼ cup mozzarella cheese and 2 tablespoons Parmesan cheese. Top with remaining 6 squares of polenta, ½ cup marinara sauce, vegetable mixture, ¼ cup mozzarella cheese and 2 tablespoons Parmesan cheese.

5. Bake 20 minutes or until cheese is melted and polenta is golden brown.

This can be done a day or two in advance.

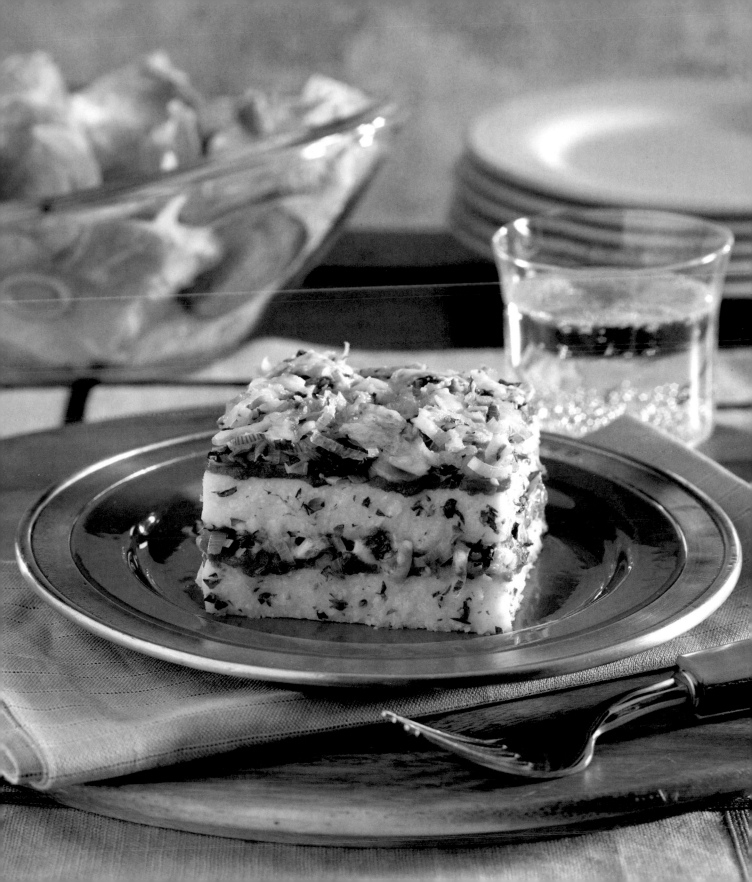

Midweek Moussaka

Makes 4 servings

1 eggplant (about 1 pound), cut into ¼-inch slices

2 tablespoons olive oil

1 pound ground beef

1 can (about 14 ounces) stewed tomatoes, drained

¼ cup dry red wine

2 tablespoons tomato paste

2 teaspoons sugar

¾ teaspoon salt

½ teaspoon dried oregano

¼ teaspoon ground cinnamon, plus additional for topping

¼ teaspoon black pepper

⅛ teaspoon ground allspice

½ (8-ounce) package cream cheese

¼ cup milk

¼ cup grated Parmesan cheese

1. Preheat broiler. Spray 8-inch square baking dish with nonstick cooking spray.

2. Line baking sheet with foil. Arrange eggplant slices on foil, overlapping slightly if necessary. Brush with oil; broil 5 to 6 inches from heat 4 minutes on each side. *Reduce oven temperature to 350°F.*

3. Meanwhile, brown beef in large nonstick skillet over medium-high heat 6 to 8 minutes, stirring to break up meat. Drain fat. Add tomatoes, wine, tomato paste, sugar, salt, oregano, ¼ teaspoon cinnamon, pepper and allspice. Bring to a boil, breaking up large pieces of tomato with spoon. Reduce heat to medium-low; cover and simmer 10 minutes.

4. Place cream cheese and milk in small microwavable bowl. Cover and microwave on HIGH 1 minute.* Stir with fork until smooth.

5. Arrange half of eggplant slices in prepared baking dish. Spoon half of meat sauce over eggplant; sprinkle with half of Parmesan cheese. Repeat layers. Spoon cream cheese mixture evenly over top. Bake 20 minutes or until top begins to crack slightly. Sprinkle lightly with additional cinnamon, if desired. Let stand 10 minutes before serving.

Or place in small saucepan over medium heat and stir until cream cheese has melted.

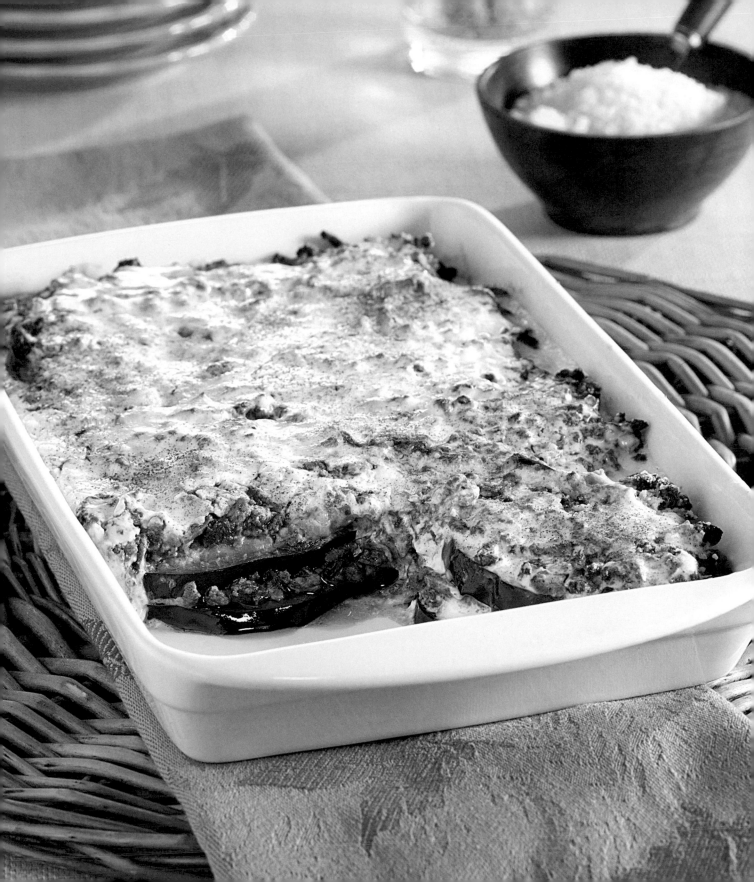

Mexican Lasagna

Makes 4 servings

1 pound ground beef

1 package (1½ ounces) gluten-free taco seasoning

1 can (about 14 ounces) Mexican-style diced tomatoes

1½ teaspoons chili powder

1 teaspoon ground cumin

½ teaspoon salt

½ teaspoon red pepper flakes

2 cups (16 ounces) sour cream

1 can (4 ounces) diced mild green chiles, drained

6 green onions, chopped

6 (8-inch) corn tortillas

1 can (15 ounces) corn, drained

2 cups (8 ounces) shredded Cheddar cheese

1. Preheat oven to 350°F. Spray 13×9-inch baking dish with nonstick cooking spray.

2. Brown beef with taco seasoning in large skillet over medium heat 6 to 8 minutes, stirring to break up meat. Drain fat.

3. Combine tomatoes, chili powder, cumin, salt and red pepper flakes in medium bowl. Combine sour cream, chiles and green onions in another medium bowl.

4. Layer one third of tomato mixture, 2 tortillas, one third of sour cream mixture, one third of meat mixture, one third of corn and one third of cheese in prepared baking dish. Repeat layers twice.

5. Bake 35 minutes or until bubbly. Let stand 15 minutes before serving.

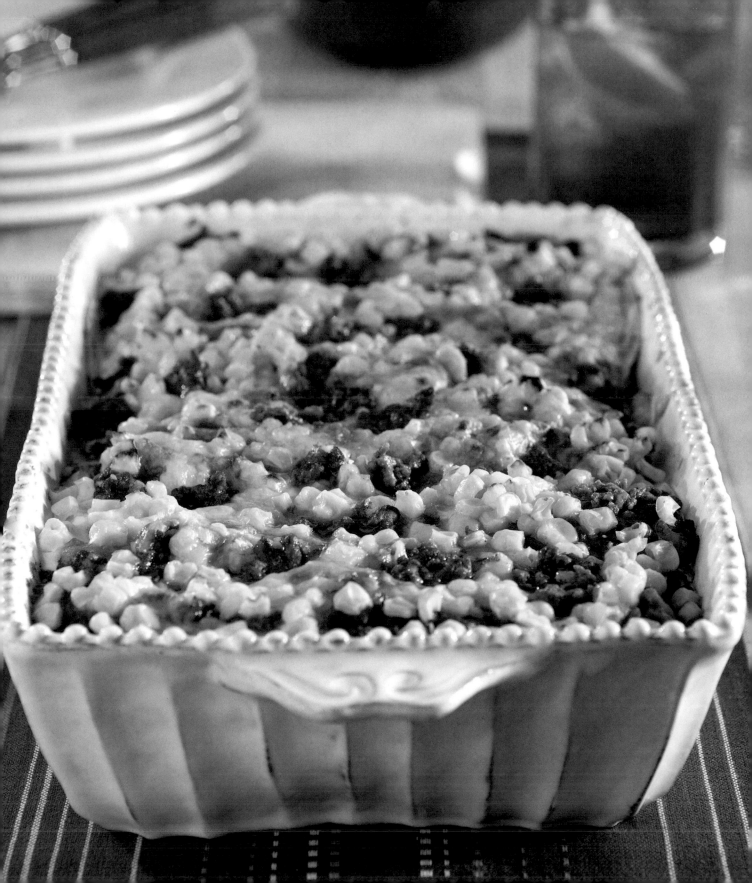

Southwest Spaghetti Squash

Makes 4 servings

1 spaghetti squash (about 3 pounds)

1 can (about 14 ounces) Mexican-style diced tomatoes

1 can (about 14 ounces) black beans, rinsed and drained

¾ cup (3 ounces) shredded Monterey Jack cheese, divided

¼ cup finely chopped fresh cilantro

1 teaspoon ground cumin

¼ teaspoon garlic salt

¼ teaspoon black pepper

1. Preheat oven to 350°F.

2. Spray baking sheet with nonstick cooking spray. Cut squash in half lengthwise; remove and discard seeds. Place squash, cut side down, on prepared baking sheet. Bake 45 minutes or just until tender. Shred squash with fork; place in large bowl. (Use oven mitts to protect hands.)

3. Add tomatoes, beans, ½ cup cheese, cilantro, cumin, garlic salt and pepper to squash; mix well.

4. Spray 1½-quart baking dish with nonstick cooking spray. Spoon squash mixture into prepared baking dish; sprinkle with remaining ¼ cup cheese.

5. Bake 30 to 35 minutes or until heated through.

Tip: The squash can be made in advance. Prepare through step 2 and store it in an airtight container in the refrigerator. Or, to save time, the squash can be cooked in the microwave. Follow the directions in the tip on page 112.

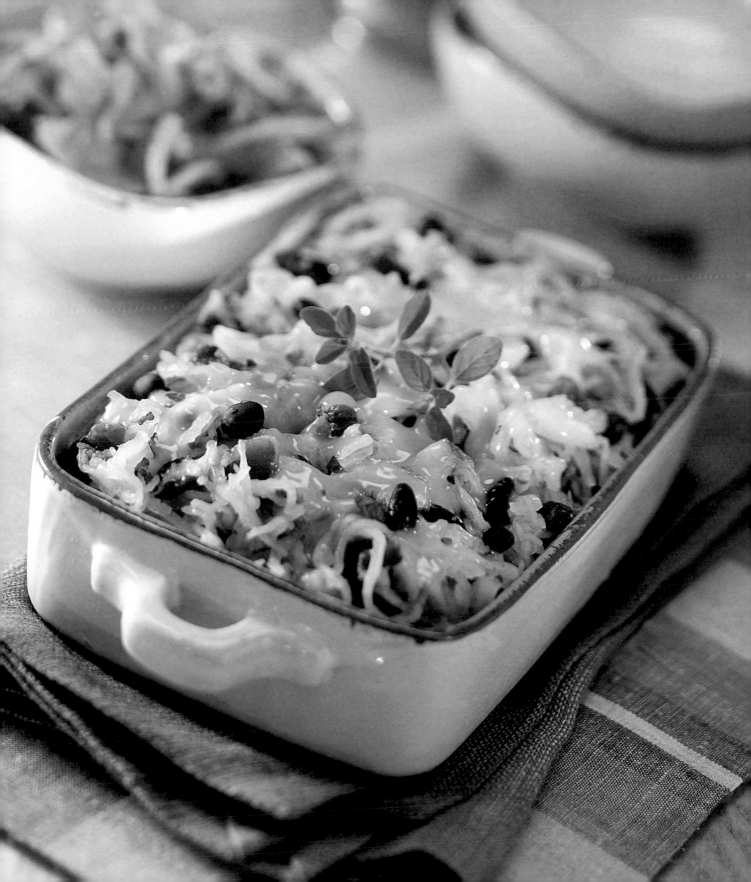

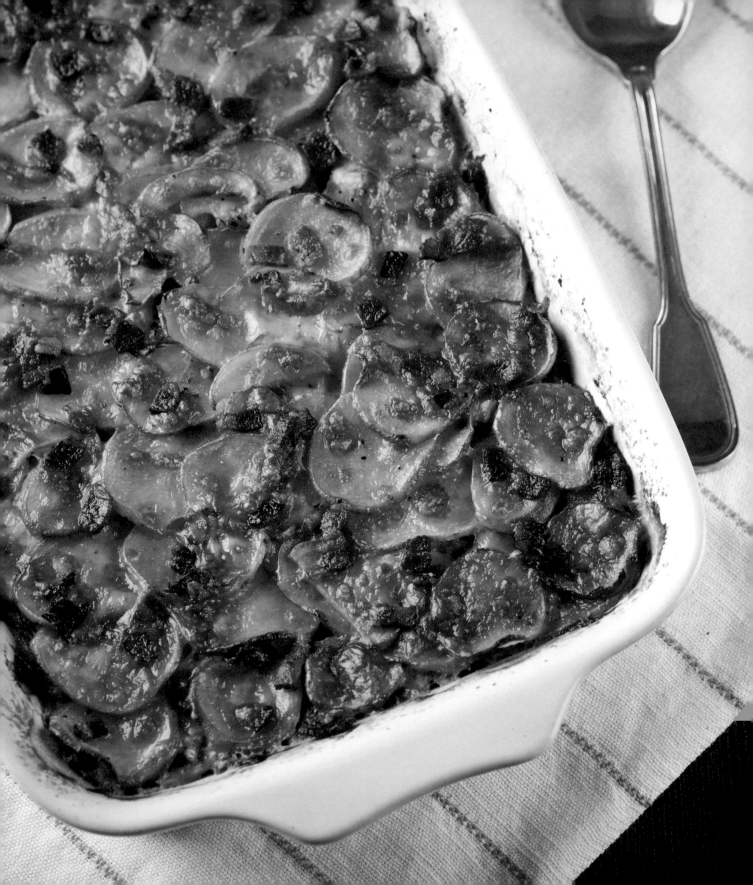

skillets *and* side dishes

Potato & Cabbage Gratin

Makes about 8 servings

1 **tablespoon butter, softened**

5 **slices bacon, chopped**

½ **head savoy cabbage, cut into ¼-inch slices (about 6 cups)**

1 **teaspoon salt, divided**

½ **teaspoon black pepper, divided**

2 **pounds peeled Yukon gold potatoes (about 12 potatoes), very thinly sliced**

3 **tablespoons cold butter, cut into small pieces**

1½ **cups (6 ounces) shredded Irish or white Cheddar cheese, divided**

¾ **cup whole milk**

1. Preheat oven to 375°F. Generously grease 2½- to 3-quart baking dish with softened butter.

2. Cook bacon in large skillet over medium-high heat until crisp. Remove to paper towel-lined plate. Drain all but 1 tablespoon drippings from skillet. Add cabbage, ¼ teaspoon salt and ⅛ teaspoon pepper to skillet; cook 12 to 15 minutes or until cabbage is crisp-tender, stirring occasionally. Reserve one third of bacon for top of gratin; stir remaining bacon into cooked cabbage.

3. Layer one third of potatoes in prepared baking dish, overlapping edges slightly. Sprinkle with ¼ teaspoon salt and ⅛ teaspoon pepper; dot with 1 tablespoon butter. Sprinkle with ½ cup cheese; top with half of cabbage mixture. Repeat layers. Top with remaining third of potatoes, ¼ teaspoon salt, ⅛ teaspoon pepper and 1 tablespoon butter. Pour milk evenly over potatoes.

4. Bake, uncovered, 30 minutes. Use flat spatula to press potatoes down into liquid. Bake 15 minutes; remove from oven and sprinkle with remaining ½ cup cheese and reserved bacon. Bake 15 minutes or until golden brown.

Pesto Zoodles & Potatoes

Makes 4 servings

3 medium red potatoes

1 large zucchini (about 12 ounces)

1 package (about 7 ounces) pesto sauce

¼ cup grated Parmesan cheese

¼ teaspoon salt

¼ teaspoon black pepper

1 cup ricotta cheese (optional)

Fresh baby arugula

1. Spiral potatoes and zucchini with fine spiral blade of spiralizer; cut into desired lengths.

2. Bring medium saucepan of salted water to a boil. Add potatoes; cook 5 to 7 minutes or until tender, adding zucchini during last 2 minutes of cooking. Drain well; return to saucepan. Stir in pesto, Parmesan cheese, salt and pepper, tossing until blended.

3. Divide zoodle mixture among four bowls. Top each serving with ricotta cheese, if desired, and serve with arugula.

Note: If you don't have a spiralizer, look for zucchini noodles in the produce section of the grocery store. Potato noodles may not be available, so try substituting another kind of vegetable noodle such as yellow squash or butternut squash instead. Or cut the potatoes into cubes or wedges and boil or roast them until tender, then toss them with the zoodles in step 2.

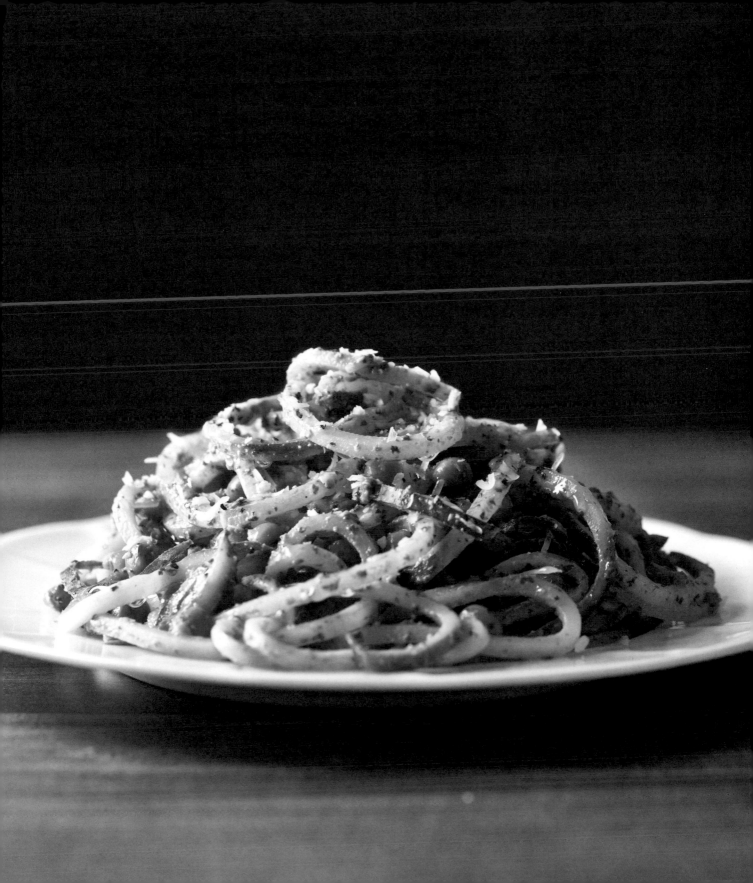

Classic Hash Browns

Makes 2 servings

1 large russet potato, peeled and grated

¼ teaspoon salt

⅛ teaspoon black pepper

2 tablespoons vegetable oil

1. Heat medium (8-inch) cast iron skillet over medium heat 5 minutes. Combine potato, salt and pepper in small bowl; toss to coat.

2. Add oil to skillet; heat 30 seconds. Spread potato mixture evenly in skillet. Cook about 5 minutes without stirring or until bottom is browned. Turn potatoes; cook 6 to 8 minutes or until golden brown and crispy.

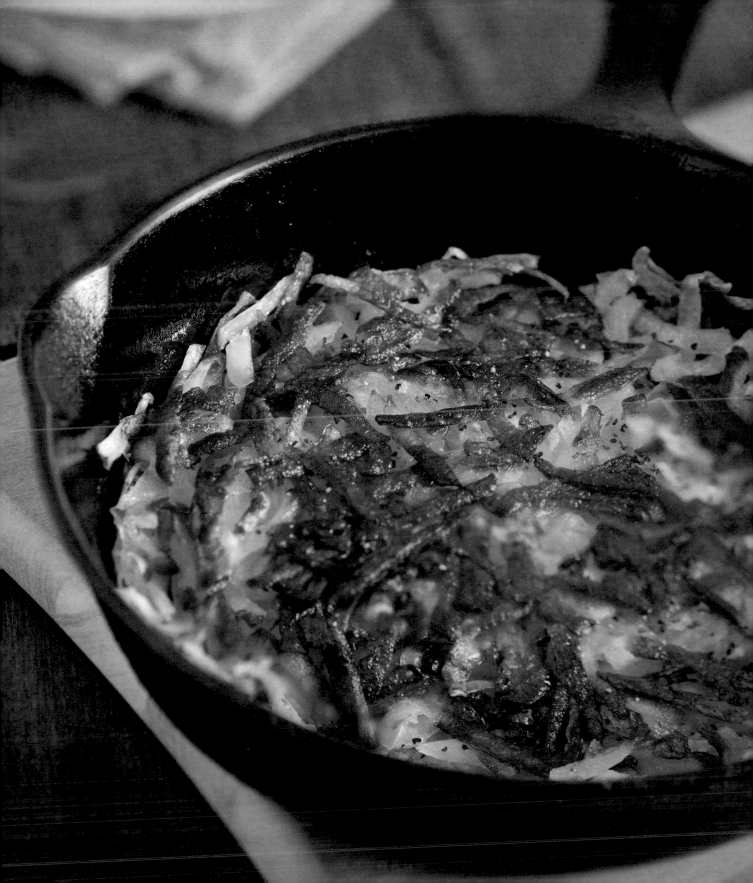

Quinoa & Roasted Corn

Makes 6 to 8 servings

1 cup uncooked quinoa

2 cups water

½ teaspoon salt

4 ears corn *or* 2 cups frozen corn

¼ cup plus 1 tablespoon vegetable oil, divided

1 cup chopped green onions, divided

1 teaspoon coarse salt

1 cup quartered grape tomatoes or chopped plum tomatoes, drained*

1 cup black beans, rinsed and drained

Juice of 1 lime (about 2 tablespoons)

¼ teaspoon grated lime peel

¼ teaspoon sugar

¼ teaspoon ground cumin

¼ teaspoon black pepper

*Place tomatoes in fine-mesh strainer and place over bowl 10 to 15 minutes.

1. Place quinoa in fine-mesh strainer; rinse well under cold running water. Combine quinoa, water and ½ teaspoon salt in medium saucepan; bring to a boil over high heat. Reduce heat to low; cover and simmer 15 to 18 minutes or until quinoa is tender and water is absorbed. Transfer to large bowl.

2. Meanwhile, remove husks and silk from corn; cut kernels off cobs. Heat ¼ cup oil in large skillet over medium-high heat. Add corn; cook 5 to 7 minutes or until tender and lightly browned, stirring occasionally. Stir in ⅔ cup green onions and coarse salt; cook and stir 1 minute. Add corn mixture to quinoa. Gently stir in tomatoes and black beans.

3. Combine lime juice, lime peel, sugar, cumin and black pepper in small bowl. Whisk in remaining 1 tablespoon oil until blended. Pour over quinoa mixture; toss lightly to coat. Sprinkle with remaining ⅓ cup green onions. Serve warm or cold.

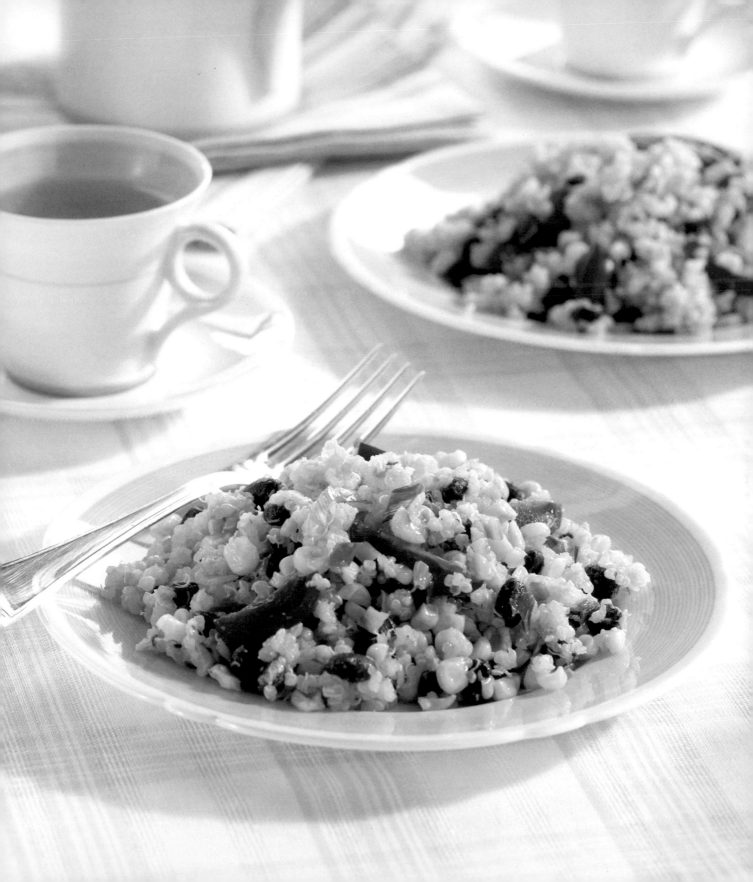

Zucchini with Toasted Chickpea Flour

Makes 4 servings

½ cup sifted chickpea flour

1½ pounds zucchini and/or summer squash (3 or 4)

2 tablespoons olive oil

1 tablespoon butter

3 teaspoons minced garlic

1 teaspoon salt

½ teaspoon black pepper

½ cup water

1. Heat large skillet over medium-high heat; add chickpea flour. Cook and stir 3 to 4 minutes or until fragrant and slightly darker in color. Remove from skillet; set aside.

2. Cut zucchini into ½-inch-thick circles or half moons. Heat oil and butter in same skillet. Add garlic; cook and stir 1 minute or until fragrant. Add zucchini, salt and pepper; cook and stir 5 minutes or until beginning to soften.

3. Stir chickpea flour into skillet to coat zucchini. Pour in water; cook and stir 2 to 3 minutes or until moist crumbs form, scraping bottom of skillet frequently to prevent sticking.

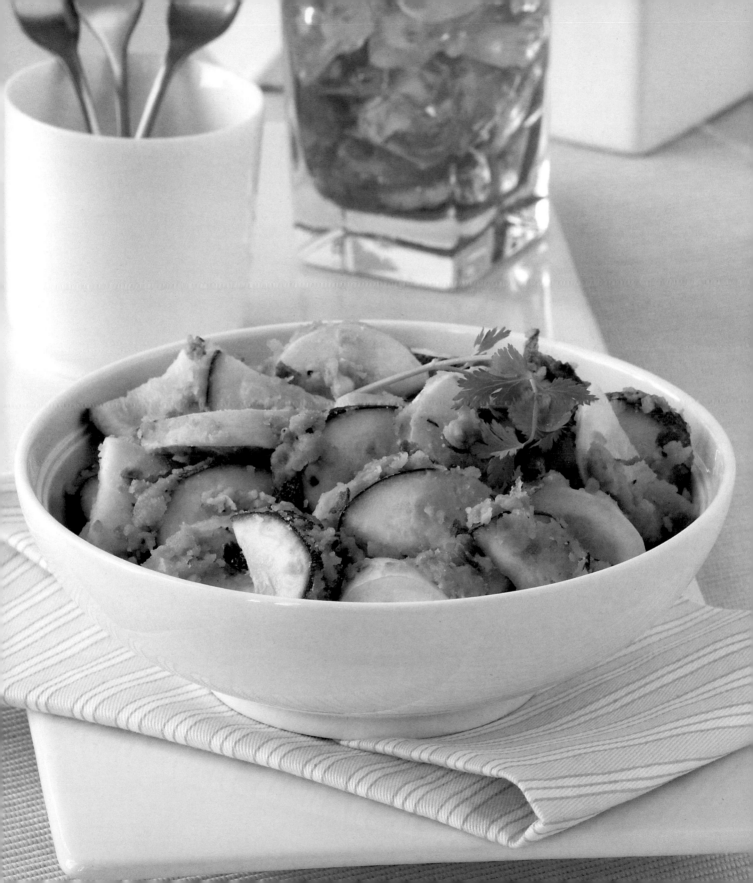

Mexican Cauliflower & Bean Skillet

Makes 4 to 6 servings

1 teaspoon olive oil

3 cups coarsely chopped cauliflower

¾ teaspoon salt

½ medium yellow onion, chopped

1 green bell pepper, chopped

1 clove garlic, minced

1 teaspoon chili powder

¾ teaspoon ground cumin

Pinch ground red pepper

1 can (about 15 ounces) black beans, rinsed and drained

1 cup (4 ounces) shredded Cheddar-Jack cheese

Salsa and sour cream

1. Heat oil in large nonstick skillet over medium-high heat. Add cauliflower and salt; cook and stir 5 minutes. Add onion, bell pepper, garlic, chili powder, cumin and ground red pepper; cook and stir 5 minutes or until cauliflower is tender. Stir in beans; cook until beans are heated through. Remove from heat.

2. Sprinkle with cheese; fold gently and let stand until melted. Serve with salsa and sour cream.

Serving Suggestion: For a hearty vegetarian main dish, serve with hot cooked brown rice and/or warm corn tortillas.

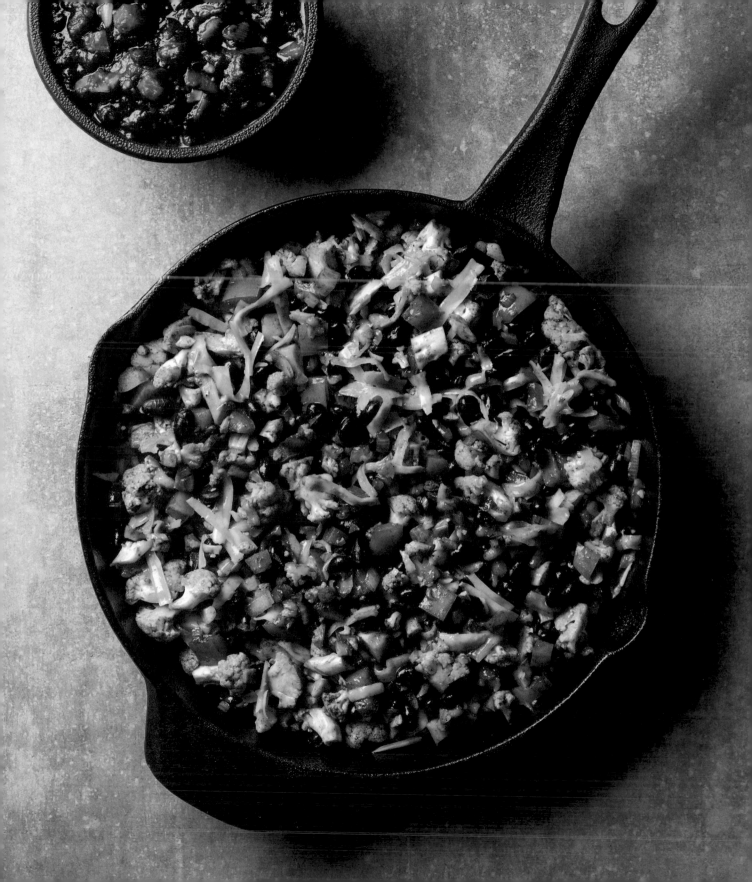

Classic Polenta

Makes 4 servings

6 cups water

2 teaspoons salt

2 cups yellow cornmeal

¼ cup vegetable oil

1. Bring water and salt to a boil in large heavy saucepan over medium-high heat. Stirring water vigorously, add cornmeal in very thin but steady stream (do not let lumps form). Reduce heat to low.

2. Cook polenta, uncovered, about 30 minutes or until thick and creamy, stirring frequently. Serve at this point for soft polenta. (See Note.)

3. For firm polenta, cook 10 to 20 minutes longer or until very thick. Polenta is ready when spoon will stand upright by itself in center of mixture. Spray 11×7-inch baking pan with nonstick cooking spray. Spread polenta evenly in baking pan. Cover; refrigerate until completely cooled and firm.

4. To serve fried, unmold polenta from baking pan onto cutting board; cut into strips or circles with round cutter.

5. Heat oil in large heavy skillet over medium-high heat; reduce heat to medium. Fry polenta pieces, half at a time, 4 to 5 minutes or until golden on all sides, turning as needed. Serve warm; garnish as desired.

Note: This versatile side dish is an important component of Northern Italian cooking and a great addition to your gluten-free cooking repertoire. The basic preparation presented here can be served in two forms. Hot freshly made polenta, prepared through step 2, can be mixed with ⅓ cup butter and ⅓ cup grated Parmesan cheese and served as a first course. Or pour onto a large platter and top with a hearty meat or vegetable sauce for a main dish. Fried polenta sticks or rounds can be served as an appetizer or as a side dish (try cutting it into fun shapes with cookie cutters for kids). Polenta shapes can also be baked, broiled or grilled.

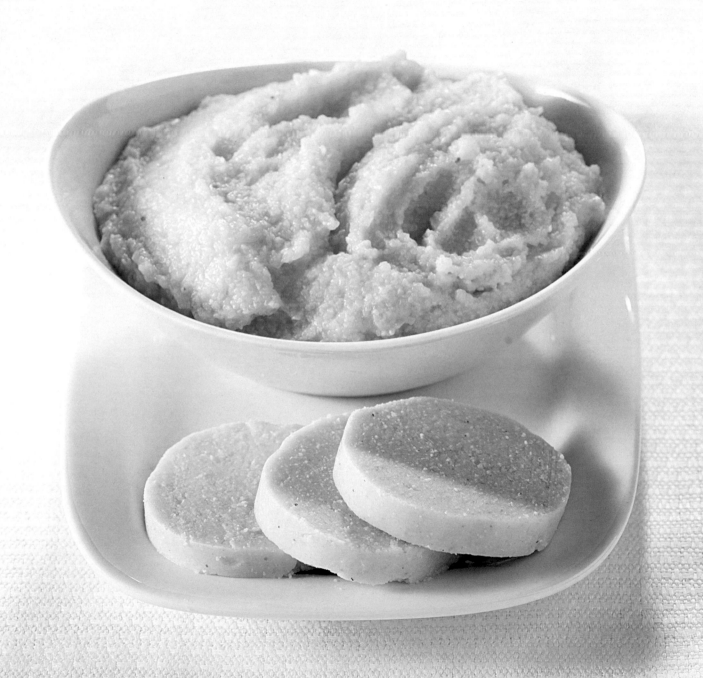

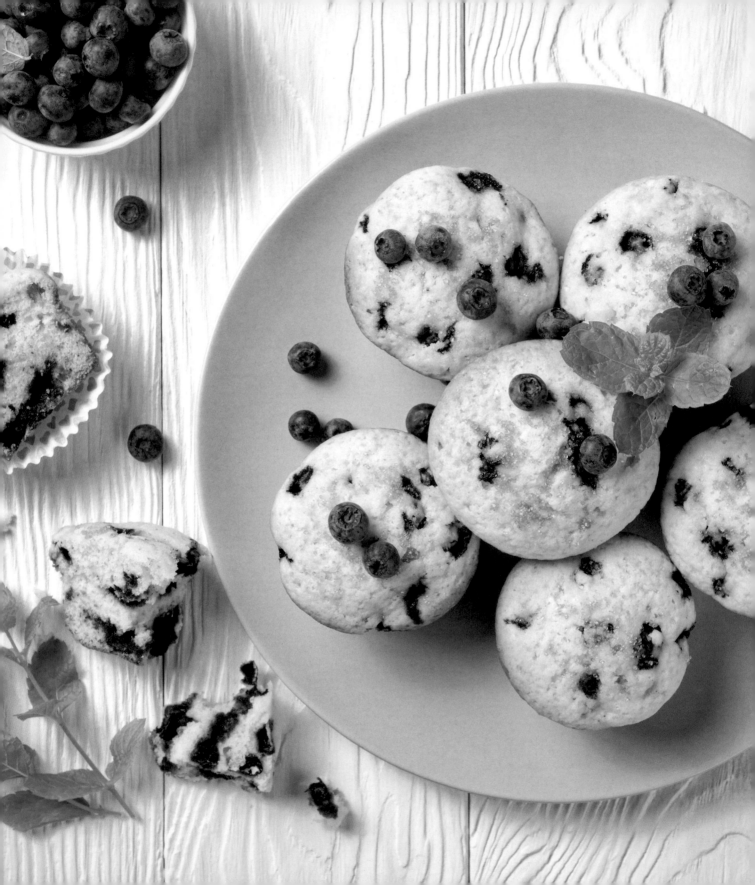

breads, muffins *and* more

Blueberry Coconut Flour Muffins

Makes 12 muffins

6 eggs

½ cup sugar

¼ cup (½ stick) butter, melted

¼ cup whole milk

½ cup plus 2 teaspoons coconut flour, divided

2 teaspoons grated lemon peel

½ teaspoon salt

½ teaspoon baking powder

½ teaspoon xanthan gum

1 cup fresh blueberries

1. Preheat oven to 375°F. Line 12 standard (2½-inch) muffin cups with paper baking cups.

2. Whisk eggs, sugar, butter and milk in medium bowl until well combined.

3. Mix ½ cup coconut flour, lemon peel, salt, baking powder and xanthan gum in medium bowl. Sift flour mixture into egg mixture. Whisk until batter is smooth.

4. Combine blueberries with remaining 2 teaspoons coconut flour in small bowl. Stir gently into batter. Divide batter evenly among prepared muffin cups.

5. Bake 12 to 15 minutes or until toothpick inserted into centers comes out clean. Cool in pan on wire rack 5 minutes. Remove from pan; serve warm.

Note: Coconut flour is a gluten-free, high-fiber, low-carbohydrate flour that adds a touch of sweetness to these muffins. Because it absorbs a great deal of liquid, a little coconut flour goes a long way. Most recipes using it also call for more eggs than usual since it can become heavy without the extra lift that eggs provide. You will find coconut flour in the specialty flour section of many supermarkets. It can also be ordered online.

Multigrain Sandwich Bread

Makes 1 loaf (about 12 servings)

1 cup brown rice flour, plus additional for pan

1¾ cups warm water (110°F)

2 tablespoons honey

1 tablespoon active dry yeast (about 1½ packages)

¾ cup white rice flour

⅔ cup dry milk powder

½ cup gluten-free oat flour

⅓ cup cornstarch

⅓ cup potato starch

¼ cup teff flour

2 teaspoons xanthan gum

2 teaspoons egg white powder

1½ teaspoons salt

1 teaspoon unflavored gelatin

2 eggs

¼ cup canola oil

1. Preheat oven to 350°F. Grease 10×5-inch loaf pan; dust with brown rice flour.

2. Combine water, honey and yeast in medium bowl; stir to dissolve yeast. Let stand 10 minutes or until foamy.

3. Combine 1 cup brown rice flour, white rice flour, milk powder, oat flour, cornstarch, potato starch, teff flour, xanthan gum, egg white powder, salt and gelatin in large bowl. Stir until well blended.

4. Whisk eggs and oil in small bowl. Gradually beat yeast mixture and egg mixture into flour mixture with electric mixer at low speed until combined. Beat at high speed 5 minutes or until smooth. Pour into prepared pan.

5. Bake 1 hour or until internal temperature reaches 200°F. Remove to wire rack; cool completely.

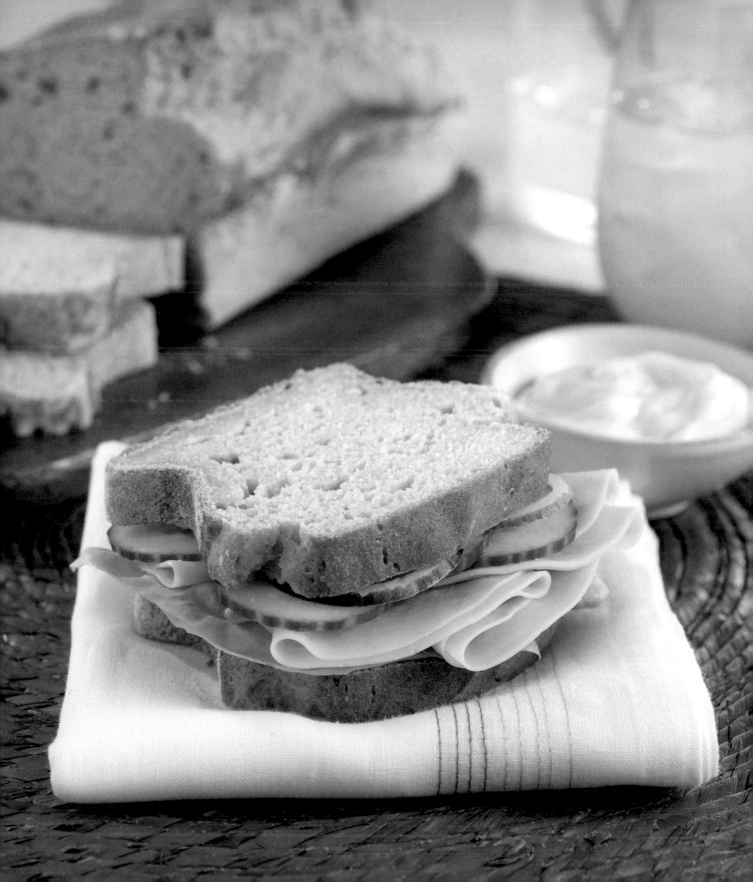

Brazilian Cheese Rolls (Pão de Queijo)

Makes about 20 rolls

1 cup whole milk

¼ cup (½ stick) butter, cut into pieces

¼ cup vegetable oil

½ teaspoon salt

2 cups plus 2 tablespoons tapioca flour*

2 eggs

1 cup grated Parmesan cheese or other firm cheese

Sometimes labeled tapioca starch.

1. Preheat oven to 350°F.

2. Combine milk, butter, oil and salt in large saucepan. Bring to a boil over medium heat, stirring to melt butter. Once mixture reaches a boil, remove from heat. Stir in tapioca flour. Mixture will be thick and stretchy.

3. Stir in eggs, one at a time, followed by cheese. Mixture will be very stiff. Cool mixture in pan until easy to handle.

4. Take heaping tablespoons of dough with tapioca-floured hands and roll into 1½-inch balls. Place on baking sheet about 1 inch apart.

5. Bake 20 to 25 minutes or until puffed and golden. Serve warm.

Note: These moist, chewy rolls are a Brazilian specialty and are always made with tapioca flour instead of wheat flour. In Brazil they are popular at breakfast, lunch or dinner.

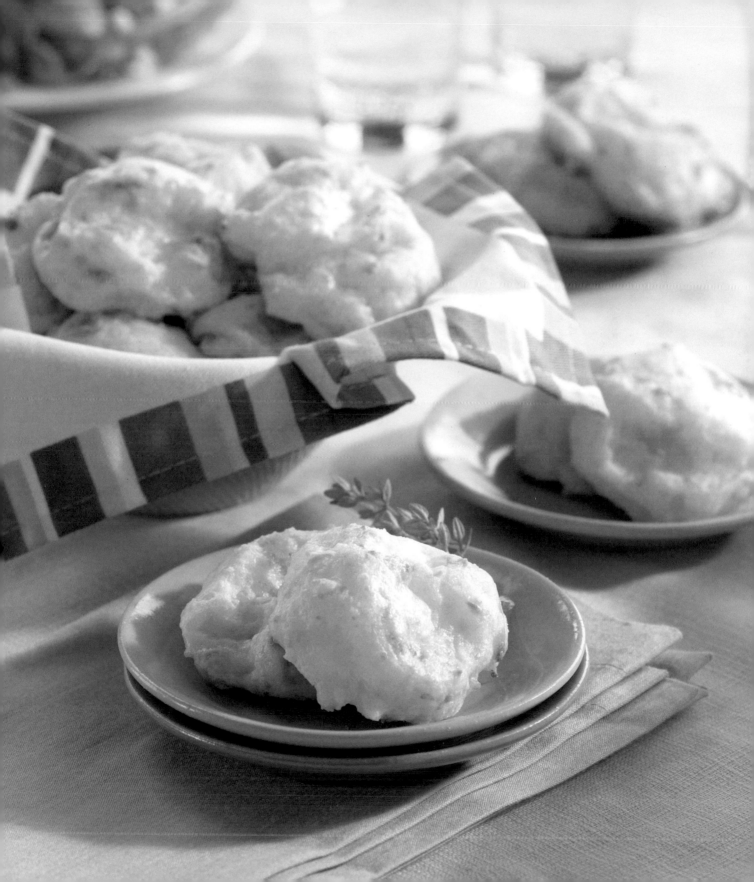

Zucchini Bread

Makes 1 loaf (about 12 servings)

3 cups one-to-one gluten-free baking flour*

⅔ cup packed brown sugar

⅓ cup granulated sugar

1 tablespoon baking powder

2 teaspoons ground cinnamon

1 teaspoon baking soda

1 teaspoon salt

¼ teaspoon ground allspice

¼ teaspoon ground nutmeg

¼ teaspoon ground cardamom

1¼ cups whole milk

2 eggs

¼ cup canola oil

1 teaspoon vanilla

1½ cups grated zucchini, squeezed dry

Or use any gluten-free all-purpose flour blend that contains xanthan gum, or make your own with the recipe on page 12.

1. Preheat oven to 350°F. Grease 9×5-inch loaf pan.

2. Combine flour, brown sugar, granulated sugar, baking powder, cinnamon, baking soda, salt, allspice, nutmeg and cardamom in large bowl; mix well. Whisk milk, eggs, oil and vanilla in medium bowl until well blended.

3. Make well in flour mixture; pour in milk mixture and stir just until blended. Stir in zucchini. Pour into prepared pan.

4. Bake 1 hour or until toothpick inserted into center comes out almost clean. Cool in pan on wire rack 5 minutes. Remove to wire rack; cool completely.

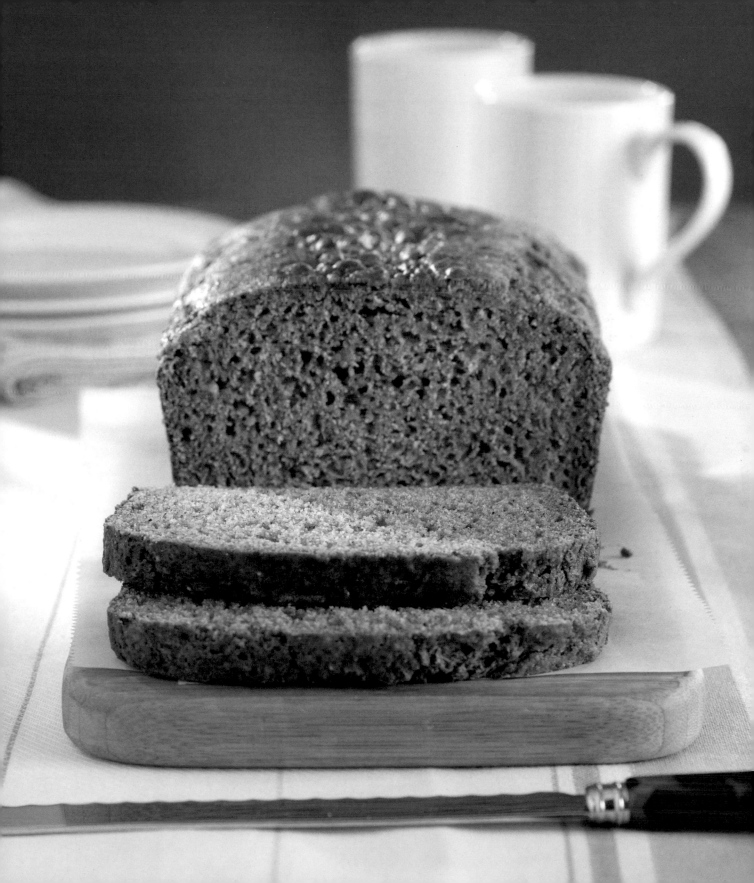

Almond Flour Quick Bread

Makes 1 loaf (16 slices)

7 tablespoons butter, divided

2 cups almond flour

3½ teaspoons baking powder

½ teaspoon salt

6 eggs, at room temperature, separated*

¼ teaspoon cream of tartar

Discard 1 egg yolk.

1. Preheat oven to 375°F. Generously grease 8×4-inch loaf pan with 1 tablespoon butter. Melt remaining 6 tablespoons butter; cool slightly.

2. Combine almond flour, baking powder and salt in medium bowl. Add melted butter and 5 egg yolks; stir until blended.

3. Place egg whites and cream of tartar in bowl of electric stand mixer; attach whip attachment to mixer. Whip egg whites at high speed 1 to 2 minutes or until stiff peaks form.

4. Stir one third of egg whites into almond flour mixture until well blended (batter will be very stiff). Gently fold in remaining egg whites until thoroughly blended (batter may look mottled). Scrape batter into prepared pan; smooth top.

5. Bake 25 to 30 minutes or until top is light brown and dry and toothpick inserted into center comes out clean. Cool in pan on wire rack 10 minutes. Remove from pan; cool completely.

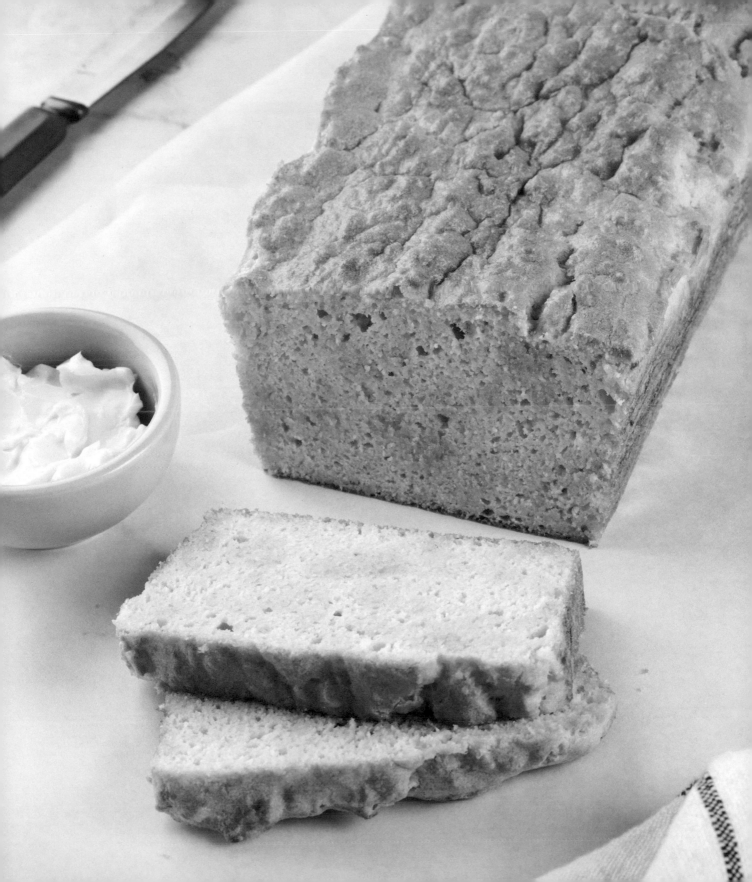

Corn Muffins

Makes 12 muffins

1 cup one-to-one gluten-free baking flour*

1 cup cornmeal

½ cup sugar

1½ teaspoons baking powder

1 teaspoon baking soda

½ teaspoon salt

1 cup buttermilk

¼ cup (½ stick) butter, melted

2 eggs

Or use any gluten-free all-purpose flour blend that contains xanthan gum, or make your own with the recipe on page 12.

1. Preheat oven to 350°F. Grease 12 standard (2½-inch) muffin cups or line with paper baking cups.

2. Combine flour, cornmeal, sugar, baking powder, baking soda and salt in large bowl. Whisk together buttermilk, butter and eggs in medium bowl. Add to dry ingredients; mix well. Batter will be thick. Spoon batter into prepared muffin cups, filling almost to top.

3. Bake 20 to 25 minutes or until lightly browned and toothpick inserted into centers comes out clean. Cool in pan 5 minutes; remove to wire rack. Serve warm.

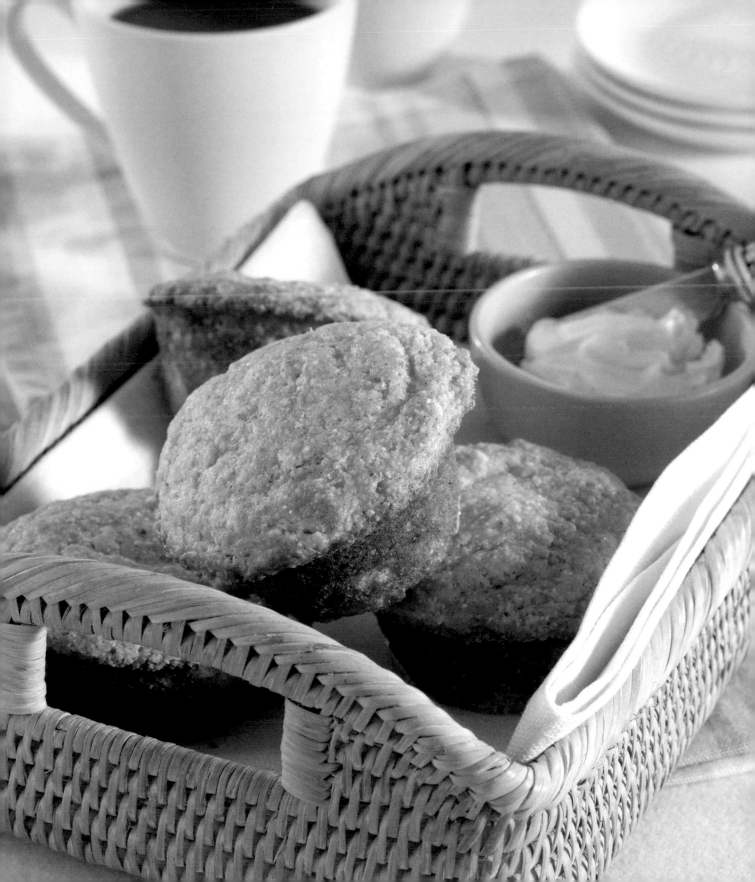

Socca (Niçoise Chickpea Pancake)

Makes 6 servings

1 cup chickpea flour

¾ teaspoon salt

½ teaspoon black pepper

1 cup water

5 tablespoons olive oil, divided

1½ teaspoons minced fresh basil *or*
    ½ teaspoon dried basil

1 teaspoon minced fresh
    rosemary *or* ¼ teaspoon
    dried rosemary

¼ teaspoon dried thyme

1. Sift chickpea flour into medium bowl. Stir in salt and pepper. Gradually whisk in water until smooth. Stir in 2 tablespoons oil. Let stand at least 30 minutes.

2. Preheat oven to 450°F. Place 9- or 10-inch cast iron skillet in oven to heat 10 minutes.

3. Add basil, rosemary and thyme to batter; whisk until smooth. Carefully remove skillet from oven. Add 2 tablespoons oil to skillet, swirling to coat pan evenly. Immediately pour in batter.

4. Bake 12 to 15 minutes or until edge of pancake begins to pull away from side of pan and center is firm. Remove from oven. Preheat broiler.

5. Brush remaining 1 tablespoon oil over top of socca. Broil 2 to 4 minutes or until dark brown in spots. Cut into wedges. Serve warm.

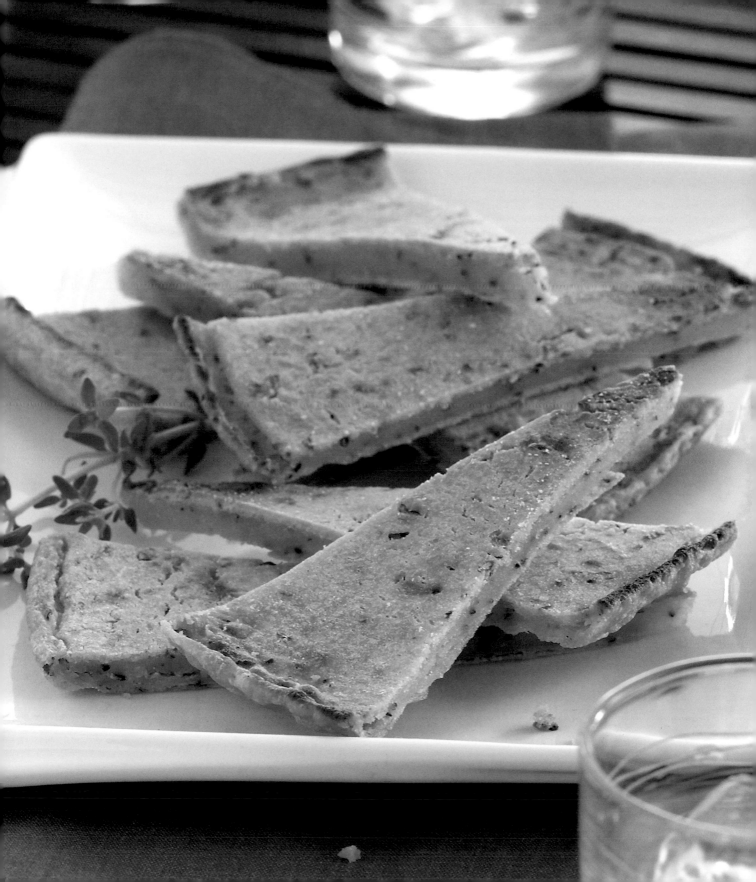

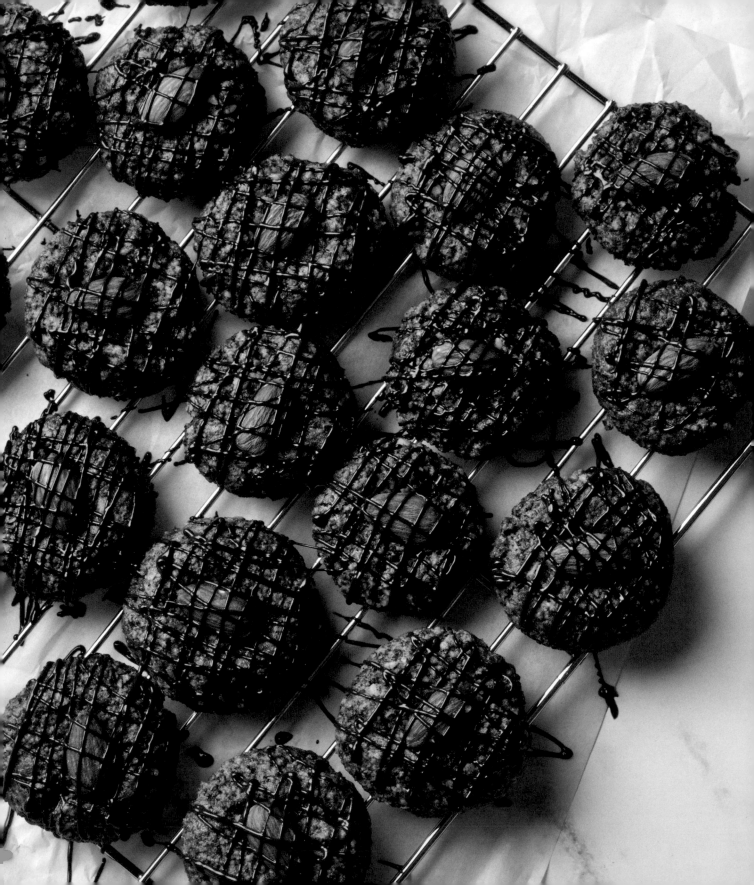

easy desserts

Mexican Chocolate Macaroons
Makes about 2 dozen cookies

8 ounces semisweet chocolate, divided

1¾ cups plus ⅓ cup whole almonds, divided

¾ cup sugar

½ teaspoon salt

2 egg whites

1 teaspoon ground cinnamon

1 teaspoon vanilla

1. Preheat oven to 400°F. Grease cookie sheets.

2. Place 5 ounces of chocolate in food processor; process until coarsely chopped. Add 1¾ cups almonds, sugar and salt; process using on/off pulses until mixture is finely ground. Add egg whites, cinnamon and vanilla; process just until mixture forms moist dough.

3. Shape dough into 1-inch balls. (Dough will be sticky.) Place 2 inches apart on prepared cookie sheets. Press 1 whole almond into center of each dough ball.

4. Bake 8 to 10 minutes or just until set. Cool on cookie sheets 2 minutes. Remove to wire racks; cool completely.

5. Chop remaining 3 ounces of chocolate. Melt in small saucepan over very low heat, stirring constantly, or place in small microwavable bowl and heat on HIGH 1 to 2 minutes, stirring at 30-second intervals until melted and smooth. Place melted chocolate in small resealable food storage bag. Cut off small corner of bag. Drizzle chocolate over cookies. Let stand until set.

Classic Brownies

Makes 2 to 3 dozen brownies

1 cup (2 sticks) butter

8 ounces semisweet baking chocolate, coarsely chopped or dark chocolate chips

1 cup sugar

4 eggs

1 teaspoon vanilla

1 teaspoon salt

1 cup one-to-one gluten-free baking flour*

¼ cup unsweetened cocoa powder

1 cup mini chocolate chips or dark chocolate chips

*Or use any gluten-free all-purpose flour blend that contains xanthan gum, or make your own with the recipe on page 12.

1. Preheat oven to 350°F. Spray 13×9-inch baking pan with nonstick cooking spray or line with parchment paper.

2. Heat butter and chocolate in large heavy saucepan over low heat; stir until melted and smooth. Remove from heat; stir in sugar until blended. Stir in eggs, one at a time, until well blended after each addition, followed by vanilla and salt. Add flour, cocoa and mini chocolate chips; stir just until blended. Spread batter evenly in prepared pan.

3. Bake 17 to 20 minutes or until center is set and toothpick inserted into center comes out clean. Cool completely in pan on wire rack. Remove from pan; cut into squares to serve.

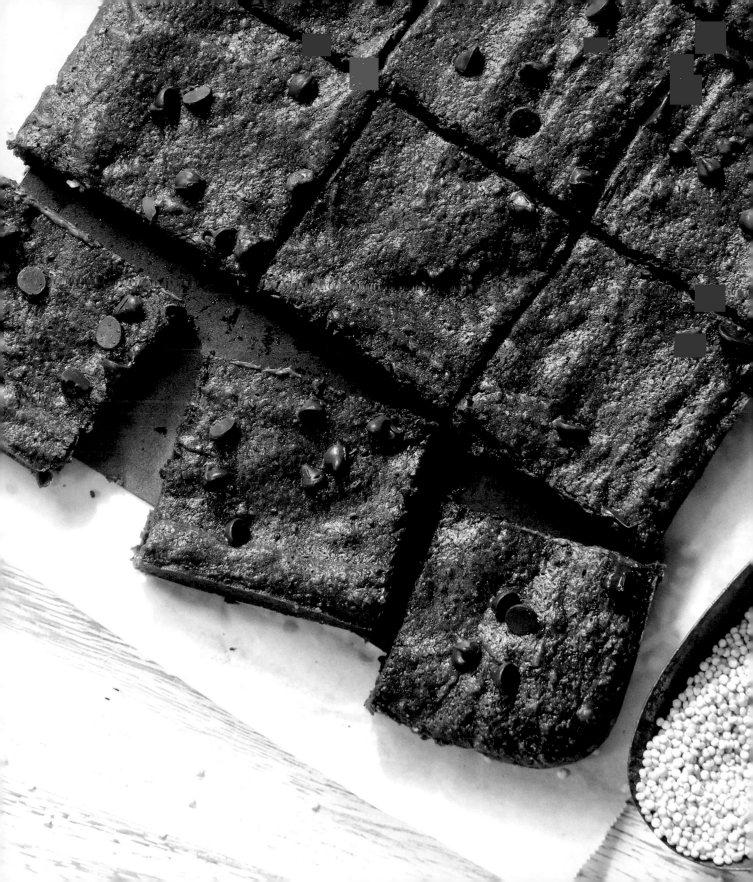

Carrot-Spice Snack Cake

Makes 8 servings

½ cup packed brown sugar

5 tablespoons butter, softened

2 eggs

½ cup milk

1 teaspoon vanilla

1¼ cups one-to-one gluten-free baking flour*

¾ cup finely shredded carrot

2 teaspoons baking powder

1½ teaspoons pumpkin pie spice

½ teaspoon salt

⅓ cup golden raisins

Powdered sugar

*Or use any gluten-free all-purpose flour blend that contains xanthan gum, or make your own with the recipe on page 12.

1. Preheat oven to 350°F. Spray 8-inch square baking pan with nonstick cooking spray.

2. Beat brown sugar and butter in medium bowl with electric mixer at medium speed until well blended. Beat in eggs, milk and vanilla.

3. Stir in flour, carrot, baking powder, pumpkin pie spice and salt. Stir in raisins.

4. Spread batter in prepared pan. Bake 25 to 30 minutes or until toothpick inserted into center comes out clean. Cool completely in pan on wire rack. Just before serving, sprinkle with powdered sugar.

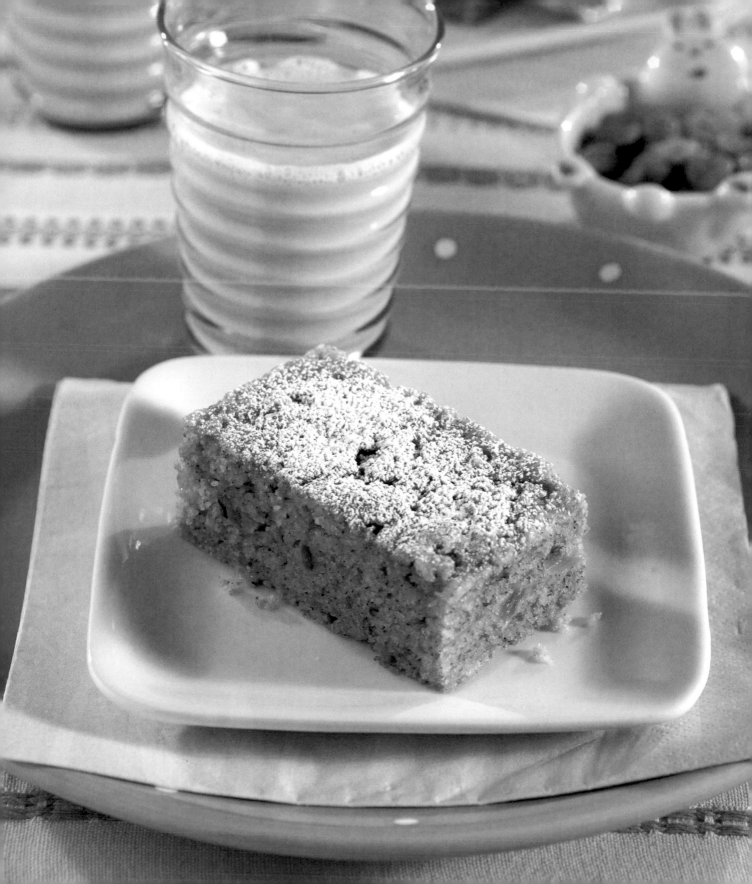

Caramel Chocolate Chunk Blondies

Makes about 2½ dozen blondies

¾ cup granulated sugar

¾ cup packed brown sugar

½ cup (1 stick) butter

2 eggs

1½ teaspoons vanilla

1 teaspoon baking powder

1 teaspoon salt

1½ cups one-to-one gluten-free baking flour*

1½ cups semisweet chocolate chunks

⅓ cup caramel ice cream topping

*Or use any gluten-free all-purpose flour blend that contains xanthan gum, or make your own with the recipe on page 12.

1. Preheat oven to 350°F. Spray 13×9-inch baking pan with nonstick cooking spray or line with parchment paper.

2. Beat granulated sugar, brown sugar and butter in large bowl with electric mixer at medium speed until smooth and creamy. Beat in eggs and vanilla until well blended. Stir in baking powder and salt. Add flour; beat at low speed until blended. Stir in chocolate chunks.

3. Spread batter evenly in prepared pan. Drop spoonfuls of caramel topping over batter; swirl into batter with knife.

4. Bake 25 minutes or until golden brown. Cool completely in pan on wire rack.

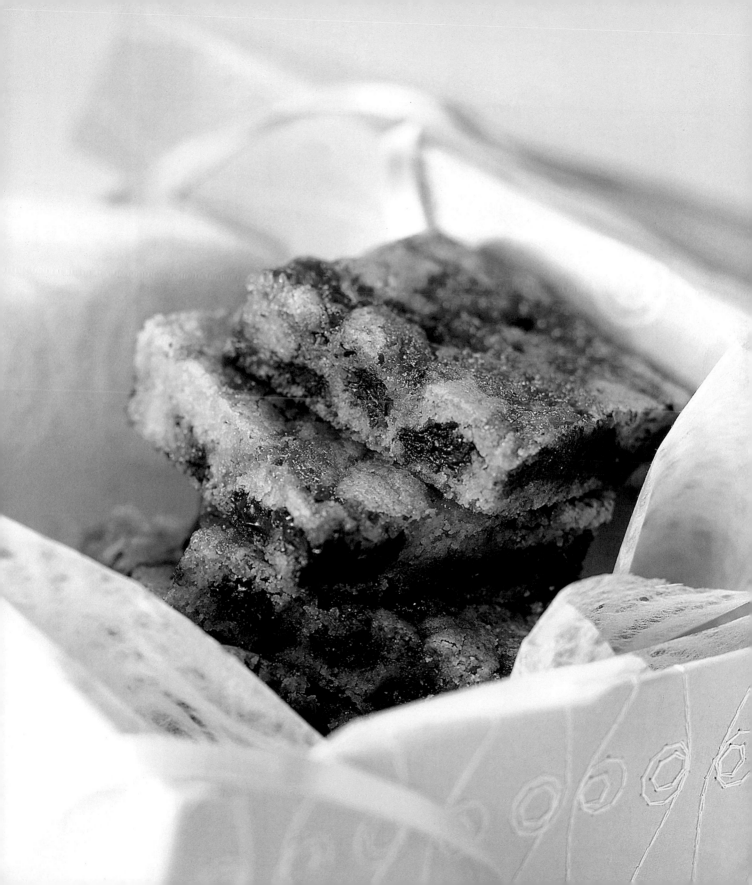

Mixed Berry Crisp

Makes about 9 servings

6 cups mixed berries, thawed if frozen

¾ cup packed brown sugar, divided

¼ cup quick-cooking tapioca

Juice of ½ lemon

1 teaspoon ground cinnamon

½ cup rice flour

6 tablespoons (¾ stick) cold butter, cut into small pieces

½ cup sliced almonds

1. Preheat oven to 375°F. Spray 8- or 9-inch square baking dish with nonstick cooking spray.

2. Combine berries, ¼ cup brown sugar, tapioca, lemon juice and cinnamon in large bowl; toss to coat. Spoon into prepared baking dish.

3. Combine rice flour, remaining ½ cup brown sugar and butter in food processor; pulse until mixture resembles coarse crumbs. Add almonds; pulse until combined. (Leave some large pieces of almonds.) Sprinkle over berry mixture.

4. Bake 20 to 30 minutes or topping is until golden brown.

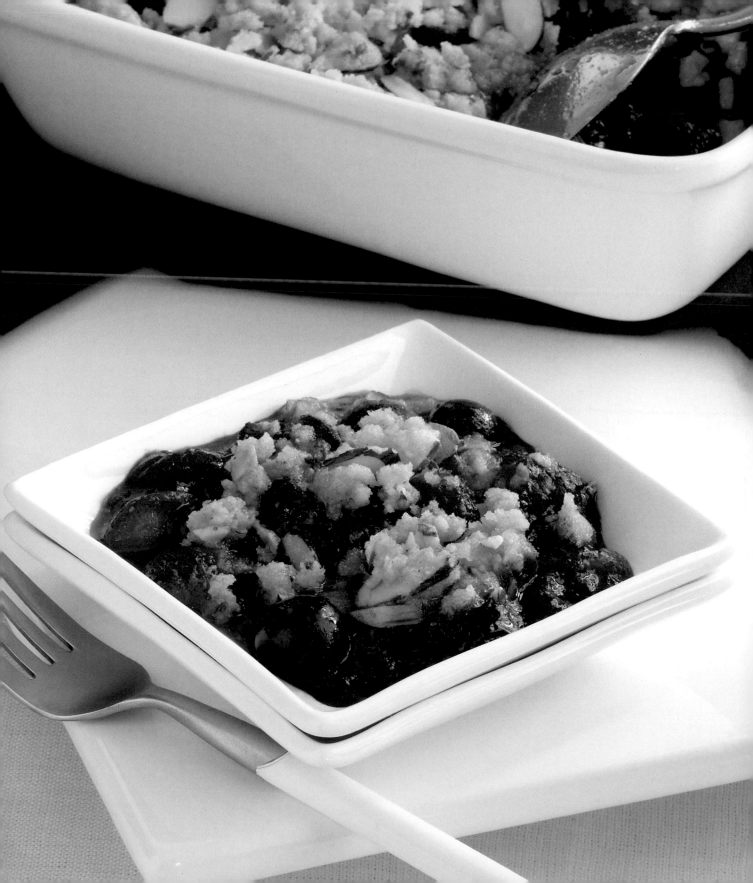

Peanut Butter Chocolate Chippers

Makes 1½ dozen cookies

1 cup packed brown sugar

1 cup creamy or chunky peanut butter*

1 egg

Granulated sugar

½ cup milk chocolate chips

Do not use natural peanut butter.

1. Preheat oven to 350°F.

2. Beat brown sugar, peanut butter and egg in medium bowl with electric mixer at medium speed until well blended.

3. Shape dough into 1½-inch balls. Place 2 inches apart on ungreased cookie sheets. Dip fork into granulated sugar; flatten each ball to ½-inch thickness, crisscrossing with fork. Press 3 to 4 chocolate chips on top of each cookie.

4. Bake 12 minutes or until just set. Cool on cookie sheets 2 minutes. Remove to wire racks; cool completely.

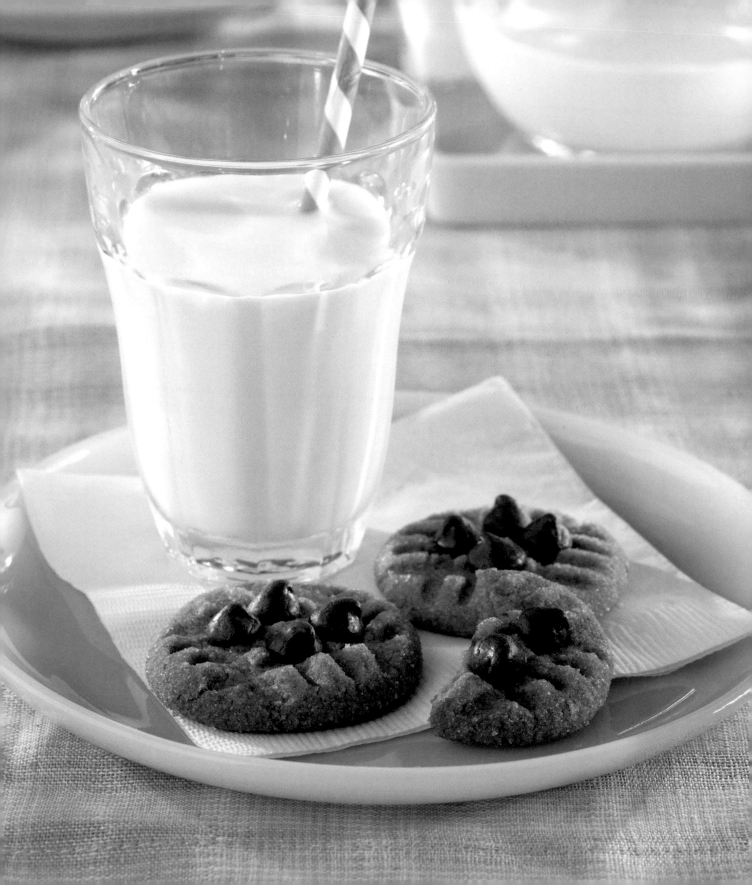

Double Chocolate Crispy Bars

Makes about 3 dozen bars

- 6 cups crisp rice cereal
- ½ cup peanut butter
- 5 tablespoons butter
- 2 ounces unsweetened chocolate
- 1 package (8 ounces) marshmallows
- 1 cup semisweet chocolate chips
- 1 cup white chocolate chips
- 2 teaspoons shortening, divided

1. Preheat oven to 350°F. Line 13×9-inch pan with waxed paper; set aside. Spread cereal on cookie sheet; toast in oven 10 minutes or until crispy; place in large bowl.

2. Meanwhile, combine peanut butter, butter and unsweetened chocolate in large heavy saucepan. Stir over low heat until chocolate is melted. Add marshmallows; stir until melted and smooth. Pour chocolate mixture over cereal; mix until evenly coated. Press firmly into prepared pan.

3. Place semisweet chocolate and 1 teaspoon shortening in medium microwavable bowl. Heat on MEDIUM-HIGH heat 1 minute; stir. Repeat heating and stirring at 10-second intervals until chocolate is melted and smooth. Spread chocolate mixture over top of bars; let stand until chocolate is set.

4. Place white chocolate and remaining 1 teaspoon shortening in separate medium microwavable bowl. Heat on MEDIUM heat 1 minute; stir. Repeat heating and stirring at 10-second intervals until chocolate is melted and smooth.

5. Turn bars out of pan onto sheet of waxed paper, chocolate side down. Remove waxed paper from bottom of bars; spread white chocolate over surface. Let stand until chocolate is set. Cut into bars.

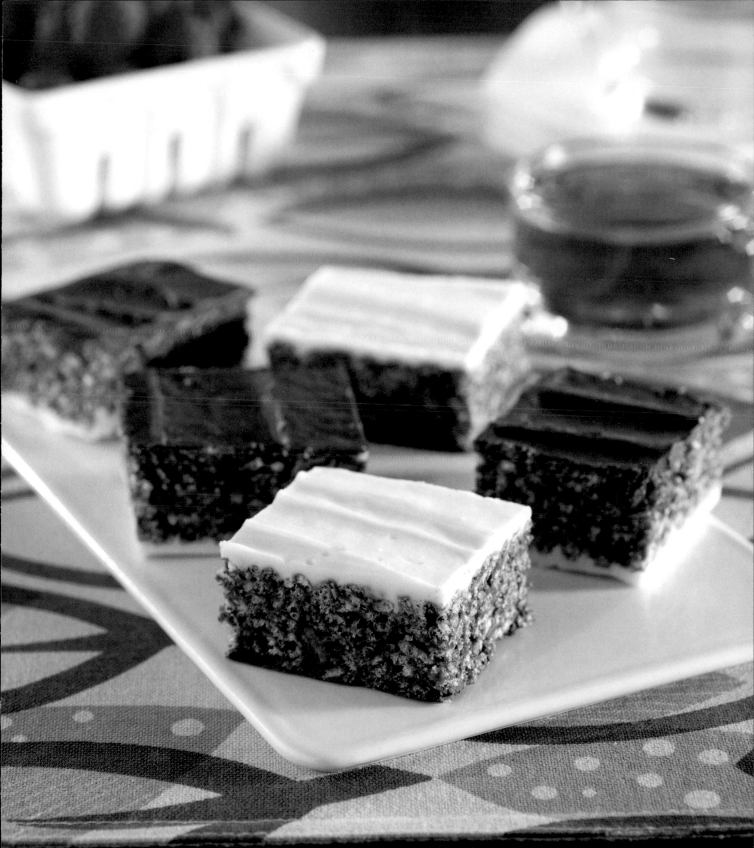

Metric Conversion Chart

VOLUME MEASUREMENTS (dry)

$^1/_8$ teaspoon = 0.5 mL
$^1/_4$ teaspoon = 1 mL
$^1/_2$ teaspoon = 2 mL
$^3/_4$ teaspoon = 4 mL
1 teaspoon = 5 mL
1 tablespoon = 15 mL
2 tablespoons = 30 mL
$^1/_4$ cup = 60 mL
$^1/_3$ cup = 75 mL
$^1/_2$ cup = 125 mL
$^2/_3$ cup = 150 mL
$^3/_4$ cup = 175 mL
1 cup = 250 mL
2 cups = 1 pint = 500 mL
3 cups = 750 mL
4 cups = 1 quart = 1 L

VOLUME MEASUREMENTS (fluid)

1 fluid ounce (2 tablespoons) = 30 mL
4 fluid ounces ($^1/_2$ cup) = 125 mL
8 fluid ounces (1 cup) = 250 mL
12 fluid ounces (1$^1/_2$ cups) = 375 mL
16 fluid ounces (2 cups) = 500 mL

WEIGHTS (mass)

$^1/_2$ ounce = 15 g
1 ounce = 30 g
3 ounces = 90 g
4 ounces = 120 g
8 ounces = 225 g
10 ounces = 285 g
12 ounces = 360 g
16 ounces = 1 pound = 450 g

DIMENSIONS

$^1/_{16}$ inch = 2 mm
$^1/_8$ inch = 3 mm
$^1/_4$ inch = 6 mm
$^1/_2$ inch = 1.5 cm
$^3/_4$ inch = 2 cm
1 inch = 2.5 cm

OVEN TEMPERATURES

250°F = 120°C
275°F = 140°C
300°F = 150°C
325°F = 160°C
350°F = 180°C
375°F = 190°C
400°F = 200°C
425°F = 220°C
450°F = 230°C

BAKING PAN SIZES

Utensil	Size in Inches/Quarts	Metric Volume	Size in Centimeters
Baking or Cake Pan (square or rectangular)	8×8×2	2 L	20×20×5
	9×9×2	2.5 L	23×23×5
	12×8×2	3 L	30×20×5
	13×9×2	3.5 L	33×23×5
Loaf Pan	8×4×3	1.5 L	20×10×7
	9×5×3	2 L	23×13×7
Round Layer Cake Pan	8×1½	1.2 L	20×4
	9×1½	1.5 L	23×4
Pie Plate	8×1¼	750 mL	20×3
	9×1¼	1 L	23×3
Baking Dish or Casserole	1 quart	1 L	—
	1½ quart	1.5 L	—
	2 quart	2 L	—